When the Patient Became a Case

Sandeep Chavan

Published by Gyrus Vision, 2026.

WHEN THE PATIENT BECAME A CASE

First edition. March 17, 2026.

ISBN: 979-8233634185

Written by Sandeep Chavan.

Table of Contents

To those who chose a profession that deals with life—and to those who expect life to be understood within it.

Medicine advances through knowledge,but it sustains through awareness.

Opening Note

This book is not written to praise doctors. Nor is it written to criticize them. It is written to pause for a moment and reflect on a profession that carries an unusual position in human society.

Medicine is not merely a career path achieved after years of study. It is one of the rare professions where knowledge, authority, and human vulnerability meet directly. A doctor does not work only with information or machines. A doctor works with uncertainty, suffering, fear, and the fragile continuity of human life.

Anyone who has passed through the demanding years of medical education knows that becoming a doctor requires far more than academic success. It demands endurance, discipline, and the ability to make decisions under pressure. These qualities deserve recognition. Yet the weight of this profession does not end with the degree. In many ways, it begins there.

Modern healthcare operates within complex systems—hospitals, regulations, insurance structures, financial pressures, and social expectations. Within this environment, doctors must balance clinical efficiency, institutional demands, and the trust placed in them by patients who arrive at their most vulnerable moments. Over time, the intensity of this environment can quietly transform how medicine is practiced and how patients are perceived.

This book invites medical professionals to step back from daily routines and examine the broader landscape in which they work. It explores how the doctor–patient relationship has evolved, how systemic pressures shape clinical practice, and why the role of a doctor extends beyond technical expertise.

Choosing medicine means choosing a profession that inevitably interacts with society's deepest concerns—health, survival, and human dignity. That responsibility does not require perfection, but it does require awareness.

The purpose of this book is not to define what a doctor should be. Rather, it is to reflect on what the profession becomes when it is practiced within complex human realities.

If this reflection prompts even a brief moment of reconsideration about the meaning of being a doctor, the purpose of these pages will have been fulfilled.

Preface

This book is not written to praise doctors.

It is not written to question their intelligence, their effort, or the years they have invested in becoming what they are.

It is written because something in modern medicine feels incomplete.

Over the years, medicine has advanced at an extraordinary pace.

Diagnosis has become sharper. Treatment has become more precise. Systems have become more organized.

And yet, in the middle of this progress, a subtle shift has taken place.

Patients are increasingly described as cases. Consultations are becoming transactions. Trust, once assumed, now has to be negotiated.

This is not a failure of medicine. It is a consequence of how medicine is being practiced within changing systems.

Doctors today operate under pressures that are rarely visible from the outside.

Long years of training reshape thinking. Institutional structures demand efficiency. Legal risks influence decisions. Time constraints compress interactions.

In such an environment, detachment becomes a survival mechanism. Standardization becomes necessary. Speed becomes unavoidable.

But survival mechanisms, if left unchecked, slowly become identity.

This book does not attempt to simplify these realities.

It does not ask doctors to be more emotional, more available, or more idealistic in a way that ignores their constraints.

Instead, it asks a more fundamental question: *What does it mean to be a doctor today?*

Not in theory. Not in tradition. But in practice—within the systems, pressures, and expectations that define modern medicine.

The purpose of this book is not to provide answers in the form of rules.

It is to create clarity.

Clarity about how medical training shapes perception. Clarity about how patients are experienced within clinical frameworks. Clarity about how systems influence behavior—often without intention.

And most importantly, clarity about the space where science and human awareness must coexist.

This is not a comfortable book.

At times, it may feel critical. At times, it may feel confronting.

That is intentional.

Because meaningful reflection rarely begins with comfort. It begins with disturbance.

If you are a doctor, this book is not asking you to change who you are.

It is asking you to observe how you practice.

To notice the small shifts that occur over time. To recognize where efficiency has replaced engagement. To see where detachment has become distance.

Not with judgment—but with awareness.

If you are willing to engage with this reflection honestly, the book will not impose a definition of a doctor on you.

It will help you define it for yourself.

Within your context. Within your system. Within your reality.

Because in the end, medicine does not lose its meaning suddenly.

It fades gradually—through small, unnoticed adjustments.

And it is restored in the same way.

Through conscious, deliberate alignment.

This book is an invitation.

Not to return to the past. But to move forward with clarity.

To practice medicine not only with knowledge, but with awareness of the human reality it serves.

The patient was never just a case.

And the doctor was never just a role.

This book exists to ensure that both are seen again—clearly.

How to Read This Book

This is not a textbook. It will not teach you how to diagnose, prescribe, or perform procedures. It does not aim to expand your clinical knowledge, nor does it compete with the science you have already mastered.

This book operates in a different space. It is written for how you practice, not what you know.

As a doctor, you are trained to read with purpose—extracting information, filtering quickly, moving toward conclusions. That approach works in clinical settings. But this book requires something else.

Do not rush through it. Each chapter is a reflection. It is meant to be read slowly, allowing you to notice not only the ideas presented, but also your own responses to them.

If something feels uncomfortable, pause there. That discomfort is intentional.

You do not need to agree with everything written here. In fact, disagreement is useful. What matters is not acceptance, but engagement.

If a section makes you question your practice, your decisions, or your interactions, then the book is doing its work.

This is not a linear argument. Some chapters may resonate deeply. Others may feel obvious, confronting, or irrelevant—until you return to them later. That is expected.

Medicine itself is not linear. Neither is reflection.

You may read this book in parts—between consultations, after a long day, or during moments of pause. It is designed to fit into the reality of your schedule, not disrupt it.

But when you read, give it your attention. Even briefly.

There are no instructions here. No checklists. No rules. Instead, there are perspectives.

Your role is to interpret them within your own context—your hospital, your specialty, your constraints, your patients.

At times, realities may feel oversimplified. At other times, they may feel stated too directly. Both reactions are valid.

This book does not attempt to capture every nuance. It attempts to highlight what is often overlooked.

If you read only intellectually, it will remain just another set of ideas. If you read reflectively, it may change how you see your practice.

There is no expectation at the end of this book. No transformation is demanded.

But if, after reading, you begin to notice—

- how you listen,
- how you speak,
- how you decide,

then something has already shifted.

That shift is enough. Because medicine does not change through large declarations. It changes through small, consistent awareness in practice.

Read this book not as a doctor seeking new knowledge, but as a practitioner willing to observe what is already happening.

That is where its value lies.

Prologue

The Day the Patient Disappeared

There was no announcement when it happened. No policy change, no declaration from a medical council, no moment that could be recorded in history. It happened quietly, almost invisibly, across hospitals, clinics, and medical schools. One day the patient was a person. Slowly, over time, the patient became a case.

This transformation did not occur because doctors stopped caring. Nor did it happen because medicine lost its scientific strength. In fact, the opposite is true. Medicine has never been more advanced. Diagnostic tools are more precise, treatment protocols more refined, and knowledge of the human body deeper than ever before.

Yet something subtle shifted in the process.

A patient no longer arrives primarily as a human story. Instead, the first interaction begins with a pattern of symptoms. Chest pain becomes a possible cardiac event. A headache becomes a neurological evaluation. Fever becomes a diagnostic pathway. The language itself changes. The patient is no longer described by who they are, but by what condition they represent.

A forty-five-year-old man with financial anxiety and sleepless nights becomes *Case 23: suspected hypertension*. A frightened young mother becomes *a post-operative recovery observation*. An elderly woman who has lived through decades of life becomes *a geriatric complication risk*.

In clinical practice this transformation is not entirely wrong. Medicine requires categorization. Without clinical classification, diagnosis would collapse into confusion. Doctors must identify patterns quickly, isolate biological causes, and move toward treatment efficiently. Precision demands abstraction.

But abstraction comes with a quiet consequence.

When a human being becomes primarily a medical case, something essential recedes into the background. The person carrying the illness becomes secondary to the illness itself. Over time, the medical mind learns to prioritize disease over experience.

Medical training gradually shapes this perception. A student enters medical school with curiosity about human life. Within a few years, the same student begins to think in clinical shorthand. This is not a flaw in education; it is a survival mechanism. Hospitals do not operate on slow philosophical reflection. They operate on decisions, protocols, and urgency.

In emergency wards, seconds matter. In intensive care units, hesitation costs lives. Doctors must learn to detach from emotional overload in order to function. A physician who absorbs every patient's fear, grief, and uncertainty would collapse under the psychological weight of the profession.

So medicine teaches a practical skill: **controlled distance**.

The doctor must see clearly without being overwhelmed. The mind must remain analytical while the situation around it may be chaotic. It is a necessary discipline. Without it, effective treatment would be impossible.

However, the same discipline that protects the doctor can slowly reshape the relationship between doctor and patient.

Over years of practice, efficiency replaces curiosity. The consultation becomes shorter. The conversation becomes more technical. The focus narrows to measurable variables: blood pressure, laboratory results, imaging findings, treatment protocols. The illness becomes clearer, but the patient becomes less visible.

At the same time, the medical system around the doctor begins to evolve in ways that reinforce this transformation.

Hospitals become institutions that must manage large volumes of patients. Time becomes a scarce resource. Administrative demands increase. Legal risks grow. Documentation expands. Insurance structures influence treatment decisions. Technology mediates interaction. Screens, reports, and digital records often stand between doctor and patient.

In such an environment, the doctor is pushed toward becoming an efficient processor of medical problems rather than a participant in human experiences.

The patient senses this shift immediately.

Many patients today do not complain about medical incompetence. Most recognize the technical expertise of modern doctors. Their frustration often lies elsewhere. They feel unheard, rushed, or reduced to numbers in a system that appears too busy to see them fully.

From the doctor's perspective, the situation looks very different.

Doctors see overcrowded waiting rooms, administrative burdens, continuous decision-making pressure, and the relentless expectation that every decision must be correct. They work within systems that demand speed, accuracy, and accountability simultaneously. What patients interpret as indifference may simply be the doctor's attempt to manage overwhelming complexity.

This is where a quiet tension develops.

Patients feel unseen. Doctors feel overburdened. Trust begins to erode on both sides.

And somewhere in this growing distance, the patient slowly disappears.

Not physically, of course. Hospitals remain full of people seeking care. But the deeper presence of the patient — the person behind the diagnosis — gradually fades from the center of medical interaction.

This book begins at that point of disappearance.

It does not claim that doctors have abandoned humanity. Such accusations are simplistic and unfair. Doctors remain among the most highly trained and dedicated professionals in society. They carry enormous responsibility, often under conditions few outside the profession fully understand.

But medicine, like any complex human system, evolves. And sometimes evolution introduces distortions that go unnoticed until they become part of everyday practice.

The question this book explores is simple, yet uncomfortable:

At what point did healing become processing?

And more importantly,

Can medicine recover the patient without losing the scientific discipline that makes modern healthcare possible?

To answer these questions, we must look carefully at the transformation that occurs when someone becomes a doctor, the pressures that shape their practice, and the expectations society places upon them.

Only then can we understand what it truly means to carry the weight of the white coat in a world where the patient is slowly disappearing — and why bringing the patient back into the center of medicine may be one of the most important responsibilities of the profession today.

PART I — BECOMING THE DOCTOR

Before a doctor begins to practice medicine, medicine has already begun to shape the doctor.

Chapter 1 — The Making of a Doctor

The First Step into Medicine

Every doctor remembers the moment the journey began, even if the memory has faded behind years of practice. It may have started as a simple aspiration during school, a family expectation, or a quiet fascination with the science of the human body. For some, it was the influence of a respected physician in the community. For others, it was the prestige attached to the profession. Regardless of the starting point, the decision to pursue medicine rarely feels ordinary. It carries the weight of ambition, responsibility, and the promise of becoming someone society deeply relies upon.

In many countries, and particularly in places like India, the path toward medicine begins long before medical school. It begins in classrooms filled with intense competition. Students spend years preparing for entrance examinations that determine whether they will be allowed to enter the world of medicine. Success is not simply a matter of interest or curiosity; it requires discipline, sacrifice, and an almost relentless focus on academic performance.

Families invest time, hope, and resources into this goal. Students reorganize their teenage years around textbooks, coaching classes, and practice tests. The idea of becoming a doctor slowly becomes more than a career choice—it becomes a defining identity long before the profession is actually reached.

By the time a student finally secures admission to medical school, the sense of achievement is enormous. It feels like crossing the first great gate toward a meaningful life. Society reinforces this feeling. A medical student is immediately seen with a certain respect, a recognition that they are preparing for a profession associated with knowledge, authority, and service.

Yet the real journey begins only after this point.

Medical school is not simply an academic program. It is an environment that reshapes the student's relationship with knowledge, time, and even with human life itself. The young student who enters the campus with curiosity and excitement soon discovers that medicine demands far more than intellectual ability. It demands endurance.

Within the first months, the scale of information becomes overwhelming. Anatomy, physiology, biochemistry, pathology—each subject opens an entirely new universe of complexity. The human body, once a familiar presence, becomes a vast map of structures, mechanisms, and interactions that must be understood with precision.

At the same time, medical education introduces the student to realities most people encounter only occasionally. Hospitals expose students to illness, suffering, and death not as distant events but as daily experiences. Patients are no longer stories heard from others; they are individuals lying in beds, waiting for diagnosis, treatment, and reassurance.

For many students, this is the first time they stand so close to the fragile boundary between life and disease.

In these early years, something important begins to change. The student gradually learns to observe the human body with scientific clarity. Symptoms must be analyzed, patterns must be recognized, and decisions must be made based on evidence rather than emotion. Curiosity slowly becomes clinical reasoning.

This transformation is necessary. Medicine cannot function on sympathy alone. It requires precision, objectivity, and disciplined thinking. But the shift from curiosity to clinical detachment is also the beginning of a deeper psychological transition.

The journey to becoming a doctor is not only about acquiring knowledge. It is about learning how to think differently, how to remain composed in difficult situations, and how to function within a profession where the consequences of decisions can be profound.

By the time the student moves deeper into medical training, the dream of becoming a doctor has already begun shaping their mind in ways they may not yet fully recognize.

The making of a doctor has begun.

1.1 — The Gate of Competition

Before a student ever steps into a medical college, the journey has already begun in a landscape defined by competition. Medicine is one of the few professions where the entry gate itself is so narrow that thousands of capable students stand outside it every year. The dream of becoming a doctor is therefore not only an academic pursuit but also a test of endurance.

For many students, this phase begins immediately after secondary school. The years that follow become intensely structured around preparation for medical entrance examinations. Coaching classes, practice tests, mock examinations, and constant evaluation become part of daily life. Time that might otherwise be spent exploring interests or enjoying youth becomes organized around a single objective: securing a seat in a medical college.

The scale of competition is enormous. In countries like India, millions of students appear for entrance examinations where only a small fraction can succeed. This reality introduces a powerful psychological shift early in the journey. Students learn that effort alone is not enough; performance must be exceptional. Precision in preparation becomes essential. Every mark carries weight.

Families often become deeply involved in this process. Parents reorganize schedules, finances, and expectations around their child's preparation. The ambition of becoming a doctor slowly becomes a shared family mission. Support, pressure, encouragement, and anxiety coexist in equal measure.

In such an environment, the student begins to experience medicine not merely as a field of study but as a *goal that demands sacrifice*. Social life shrinks. Recreational activities become rare. Conversations with friends frequently revolve around ranks, scores, and exam strategies. Success or failure is measured by a number printed on a results sheet.

This stage shapes the mindset of future doctors in important ways.

First, it teaches discipline. Students learn to focus intensely for long periods, to handle complex information, and to work under pressure. These abilities later become valuable in medical training and clinical practice.

Second, it introduces the habit of *thinking competitively*. The student becomes accustomed to measuring progress relative to others. Medicine begins as a collaborative profession, but its entry is defined by rivalry. Only those who remain among the highest performers move forward.

Third, it establishes an early association between medicine and *achievement*. Securing admission to a medical college becomes a moment of immense validation—not only academically but socially. The student who enters medical school is often celebrated within family and community. Respect arrives even before the profession has actually begun.

Yet the Gate of Competition also leaves subtle marks.

Years of intense preparation can narrow intellectual curiosity. Learning becomes strongly exam-oriented. The student becomes skilled at solving problems and remembering details but may have had little time to reflect on the deeper human dimensions of medicine. Questions such as *what it means to treat people, how illness affects families*, or *how doctors carry responsibility* often remain distant during this stage.

At this point, medicine still appears primarily as a destination.

The student believes that once the entrance exam is cleared and the medical college secured, the difficult part of the journey has ended. In reality, the competition was only the first filter. The true transformation of the student into a doctor has not yet begun.

The gates have opened—but the path ahead is far more demanding than the student yet realizes.

1.2 — The Years of Immersion

Once the gate of competition has been crossed and the student enters medical school, a new phase begins—one that is less visible to the outside world but far more transformative. If the entrance examination tested determination, medical education now tests endurance.

For many students, the first weeks in medical school bring a mixture of excitement and quiet shock. The scale of knowledge is overwhelming. Subjects that were once briefly introduced in school suddenly expand into vast domains of study. Anatomy alone demands an understanding of hundreds of structures, pathways, and relationships inside the human body. Physiology introduces complex mechanisms governing life itself. Biochemistry reveals intricate molecular interactions that sustain every cell.

The student quickly realizes that medicine is not simply about learning facts; it is about understanding systems that operate simultaneously and continuously within the body.

Days begin early and often end late. Lectures, laboratory sessions, practical examinations, and self-study fill most waking hours. The schedule leaves little room for casual learning or slow reflection. Medical education moves with urgency because the volume of information is immense and the responsibility attached to that knowledge is serious.

One of the most powerful moments during these years occurs in the anatomy laboratory. For many students, it is their first direct encounter with the human body as an object of scientific study. Standing beside a cadaver, the student confronts a profound reality: the human body is no longer an abstract concept from textbooks. It is tangible, complex, and deserving of careful respect.

The anatomy lab silently teaches several lessons at once. It teaches precision, because every structure has a location and function that must be understood clearly. It teaches humility, because the complexity of the body quickly reveals the limits of superficial knowledge. And it teaches a quiet gratitude toward those who allowed their bodies to become instruments of medical learning.

As the years progress, medical education expands beyond classrooms and laboratories into hospital wards. Clinical postings introduce students to patients who are living through illness rather than studying it. Symptoms described in textbooks now appear in real human beings, each with a unique story, background, and emotional response to disease.

This is often the first time students begin to observe the human side of medicine closely.

They see anxiety in a patient waiting for test results. They watch families sit quietly beside hospital beds. They witness pain, recovery, disappointment, and sometimes death. These experiences can be deeply moving, especially in the early stages when the student has not yet developed the emotional distance that experienced doctors often maintain.

At the same time, the student begins learning the language of clinical reasoning. Conversations between doctors focus on diagnosis, laboratory findings, imaging results, and treatment plans.

Patients are discussed through medical terminology that allows professionals to communicate quickly and precisely.

Gradually, the student learns to shift between two perspectives: seeing the patient as a person and understanding the illness as a clinical condition. Balancing these perspectives becomes one of the subtle challenges of medical training.

During these years, another change quietly occurs. Medicine begins to occupy the center of the student's life. Academic responsibilities leave little space for other pursuits. The identity of the student becomes increasingly tied to the profession they are preparing to enter.

Friends outside medicine often follow different schedules and concerns. Conversations begin to revolve around clinical cases, examinations, hospital experiences, and future specializations. Slowly, the world of medicine becomes its own environment with its own rhythms, pressures, and expectations.

This period of immersion is demanding but necessary. Without deep exposure to knowledge, patients, and clinical environments, the student cannot develop the competence required for responsible medical practice.

Yet these years also shape the psychological foundation of the future doctor. The student learns to absorb large amounts of information, to remain focused under pressure, and to adapt to a life where the boundaries between study, work, and responsibility often blur.

By the time the student moves further into clinical training, medicine is no longer simply something they study. It becomes the lens through which they begin to see the human body—and eventually, the human being.

1.3 — The Hierarchy of Medicine

Every profession has its structure, but medicine operates within one of the most defined hierarchies in the professional world. From the moment a student enters medical training, they become part of a system where authority, responsibility, and experience are clearly layered.

At the top stand senior professors and consultants—individuals who have spent decades studying, practicing, and teaching medicine. Below them are associate professors, assistant professors, senior residents, junior residents, interns, and finally medical students. Each level carries its own responsibilities, privileges, and expectations.

For a new student entering the system, this hierarchy becomes immediately visible. Knowledge in medicine is not only transferred through textbooks; it is transmitted through observation, correction, and disciplined practice under supervision. Students learn by watching how senior doctors interact with patients, how they make clinical decisions, and how they respond in moments of uncertainty.

The hierarchy ensures order in an environment where mistakes can have serious consequences. Decisions about diagnosis and treatment must follow clear lines of responsibility. A student observes, an intern assists, a resident manages cases under supervision, and a consultant ultimately carries the final authority. This structure protects patients while allowing younger doctors to learn gradually.

Yet the hierarchical nature of medicine also shapes the personality of those moving through it.

Young medical students quickly learn the importance of discipline and humility. Questions must be asked carefully, instructions followed precisely, and mistakes corrected immediately. Clinical rounds often become moments of intense learning where senior doctors test the knowledge of trainees. A student presenting a case must recall details accurately, interpret symptoms correctly, and defend clinical reasoning.

These experiences can be both intimidating and transformative.

Under pressure, students develop mental sharpness. They learn to organize information quickly, think logically, and speak with clarity. Medicine rewards those who can maintain composure while being questioned or challenged.

However, the hierarchical culture can also introduce certain tensions. Long-standing traditions in medical training sometimes blur the line between rigorous teaching and excessive pressure. Senior doctors, having passed through demanding training themselves, may expect the same level of endurance from younger trainees.

This culture often reinforces an unspoken rule within medicine: *resilience is assumed, not explained.*

Students and junior doctors adapt by becoming tougher. Emotional sensitivity gradually becomes secondary to professional competence. The ability to absorb criticism without hesitation becomes part of professional survival.

Within this structure, respect flows both ways when the system functions well. Senior doctors guide younger ones through complex medical situations, sharing insights that cannot be found in textbooks. Trainees, in turn, contribute energy, effort, and continuous learning to the healthcare system.

But hierarchy also quietly teaches another lesson: *medicine is not practiced in isolation*. Every doctor operates within a chain of responsibility that extends beyond the individual. Decisions are influenced by experience, institutional protocols, and the collective wisdom of the profession.

For the student moving through this structure, medicine becomes more than a body of knowledge. It becomes a disciplined culture shaped by generations of practitioners.

By the time the young trainee begins handling patients more independently, the hierarchy that once felt intimidating begins to feel familiar. The student who once stood quietly at the edge of clinical rounds now finds themselves presenting cases, making decisions, and guiding those who are just entering the system.

In this way, the hierarchy of medicine does more than organize learning. It slowly prepares the student to step into authority—a position where knowledge must eventually transform into responsibility.

1.4 — The First Encounters with Reality

Until a certain point in medical education, illness exists primarily inside textbooks. Diseases are described through diagrams, classifications, and carefully written case descriptions. Symptoms appear as bullet points. Treatment protocols are structured, logical, and neatly organized. In this environment, the study of medicine feels systematic and intellectually manageable.

The first clinical exposure changes that perception permanently.

When medical students begin their ward postings, they step into an environment where illness is no longer theoretical. The hospital is not a classroom; it is a living system filled with uncertainty, urgency, and human vulnerability. The patient in the hospital bed is not a hypothetical case but a person experiencing real pain, fear, and hope.

For many students, the first patient examination becomes a defining moment.

Standing beside the bed, the student introduces themselves, often with a mixture of curiosity and nervousness. They begin asking questions—about symptoms, duration of illness, past medical history. These questions follow patterns learned in lectures, yet the conversation often unfolds unpredictably. Patients speak about discomfort, worries about family, financial stress, and anxieties about their future. Illness rarely appears as a clean narrative.

At this moment, the student begins to realize something that textbooks cannot fully convey: disease does not exist independently of the person experiencing it.

The first clinical encounters also introduce students to situations that can be emotionally unsettling. A patient may cry while describing their pain. A family member may ask questions the student cannot answer. A critically ill patient may be surrounded by worried relatives searching for reassurance. In such moments, the student becomes aware that medicine involves not only knowledge but also the management of human expectations.

Among the most profound experiences for many trainees is witnessing death for the first time in a clinical setting.

In everyday life, death is often distant or private. In hospitals, it can be sudden and immediate. Students observe doctors attempting resuscitation, adjusting medications, and making rapid decisions while time moves relentlessly forward. Despite all efforts, there are moments when medicine reaches its limits.

For a young trainee, these moments can be deeply sobering.

They reveal that medicine, despite its power, does not control life completely. The doctor's role includes not only curing but also managing uncertainty and sometimes accepting outcomes that cannot be reversed.

These early experiences begin shaping the emotional landscape of the future doctor.

At first, many students react with strong empathy. They feel the patient's suffering intensely and may carry those emotions long after leaving the hospital. However, repeated exposure to illness gradually requires the development of emotional boundaries. Without some level of psychological distance, the emotional weight of clinical practice would become overwhelming.

This is where a subtle transformation begins.

The student learns to focus on clinical details even when situations are emotionally charged. Attention shifts toward measurable signs—vital parameters, laboratory values, imaging results. Clinical reasoning becomes the primary guide for action. Compassion does not disappear, but it begins to operate within a more structured mental framework.

This adaptation is neither entirely good nor entirely bad. It is part of learning how to function effectively in medicine.

Yet these first encounters with reality leave lasting impressions. They remind the student that every disease carries a human story and that every medical decision affects not just a body but a life surrounded by relationships, responsibilities, and hopes.

As clinical exposure increases, the student gradually becomes more confident. Conversations with patients become smoother. The hospital environment becomes familiar. The uncertainty that once felt intimidating begins to feel manageable.

But something else is also taking shape quietly during these years.

The student who entered medical school with curiosity about the human body is now beginning to see illness through a professional lens. Patterns replace surprises. Clinical categories replace narratives. Medicine slowly organizes reality into forms that can be understood, diagnosed, and treated.

The process is essential for becoming a doctor.

Yet it also marks the beginning of a deeper transformation—the gradual shift from observing people with illness to analyzing illness within people.

1.5 — Exhaustion as a Teacher

If the early years of medical education introduce knowledge and clinical exposure, the later stages—particularly internship and residency—introduce something far more demanding: responsibility under exhaustion.

This phase of training is often where the idealism of becoming a doctor meets the operational reality of medicine.

Young doctors suddenly find themselves inside a system that runs continuously. Hospitals do not follow normal working hours. Illness does not wait for convenience. Emergencies arrive at midnight, complications appear without warning, and decisions often must be made quickly with limited time and information.

Interns and residents become the frontline workforce of this system.

Long shifts become routine. Night duties extend into early mornings. Sleep becomes irregular and often insufficient. A resident may move from one ward to another, responding to calls, reviewing patient charts, writing notes, assisting procedures, and preparing case discussions for senior doctors.

For many trainees, this period is physically and mentally exhausting.

Yet exhaustion is not treated as an obstacle within medical culture. It is almost accepted as a natural part of professional development. The reasoning behind this tradition is practical: doctors must learn to function under pressure because clinical situations rarely provide comfortable conditions.

In emergency medicine, intensive care, and surgical environments, the ability to remain focused despite fatigue can mean the difference between effective treatment and dangerous delay. Training therefore exposes young doctors to demanding situations so they can develop resilience.

However, the intensity of this period reshapes the trainee in several ways.

First, decision-making becomes faster and more instinctive. Residents gradually develop clinical intuition—the ability to recognize patterns quickly and respond appropriately. A patient's subtle change in condition, a slight variation in vital signs, or an unusual symptom may trigger immediate action because the doctor has learned to recognize warning signals.

Second, responsibility becomes real.

During earlier years of training, students observe and assist. During residency, the young doctor often becomes directly involved in patient management. They write orders, adjust treatments, and communicate updates to senior doctors. The consequences of these decisions are no longer theoretical.

This responsibility can be both empowering and intimidating. Every young doctor remembers the first time they realize that a patient's progress depends partly on their judgment.

Third, emotional endurance becomes essential.

Residency exposes doctors repeatedly to situations where outcomes are uncertain. Some patients recover quickly. Others deteriorate despite careful treatment. The young doctor learns that medicine does not always provide satisfying conclusions. Sometimes the best possible care still leads to loss.

Under such circumstances, exhaustion interacts with emotional pressure. The doctor must continue working even after difficult cases, because the hospital environment never pauses.

Over time, a particular mindset begins to develop. The young doctor learns to compartmentalize experiences—placing difficult emotions aside temporarily in order to continue functioning. Clinical focus becomes the primary tool for maintaining stability.

This adaptation allows doctors to survive demanding environments. Without it, the emotional and physical strain of medical practice would quickly become unbearable.

But exhaustion also teaches another lesson.

It reveals the limits of human capacity.

Young doctors realize that medicine is not performed by flawless individuals. It is practiced by human beings who must constantly balance fatigue, responsibility, and complex decisions. The myth of the tireless doctor slowly fades, replaced by the reality of a profession that demands extraordinary stamina.

At the same time, this period strengthens a deep professional bond among those undergoing similar training. Interns and residents share experiences that few outside the profession fully understand—long nights, critical cases, unexpected recoveries, and difficult losses. These shared moments create a sense of solidarity within the medical community.

By the time residency approaches its later stages, the young doctor has changed significantly from the student who once entered medical school with excitement and uncertainty.

Knowledge has expanded. Clinical judgment has sharpened. Responsibility has become familiar.

And somewhere within this transformation, exhaustion has quietly played the role of an unspoken teacher—forcing the doctor to discover how much pressure the profession truly demands.

1.6 — The Psychological Reshaping

By the time a medical student advances through years of study, clinical exposure, and demanding training, something deeper than knowledge has changed. The transformation is not limited to what the doctor knows—it extends to how the doctor thinks, observes, and interprets human life.

Medical education gradually reshapes perception itself.

In the beginning, the student approaches patients with curiosity and a natural emotional response. Illness appears dramatic, suffering feels intense, and every case seems unique. But as clinical experience accumulates, the mind begins to organize these experiences into recognizable patterns.

A cough is no longer simply a complaint; it becomes a possible respiratory condition. Abdominal pain becomes a differential diagnosis. Fever triggers a systematic search for infection or inflammation. What once appeared as scattered symptoms now fit into structured medical frameworks.

This shift is essential for the practice of medicine.

Doctors cannot rely solely on emotional interpretation. Clinical reasoning requires the ability to categorize information, identify patterns, and make decisions based on probabilities rather than impressions. The medical mind learns to filter vast amounts of information and focus on the details that matter most for diagnosis and treatment.

Over time, this process becomes almost automatic.

A trained physician entering a ward does not merely see people resting in beds. The physician sees vital signs, laboratory reports, treatment progress, risk factors, and potential complications. Each patient becomes a dynamic medical situation requiring monitoring and interpretation.

In many ways, this transformation represents the development of professional intelligence. It allows doctors to navigate complex clinical situations efficiently. Without such structured thinking, medicine would become chaotic and unreliable.

However, the same transformation introduces a subtle psychological distance.

As clinical thinking strengthens, emotional responses often become more controlled. Doctors learn to manage reactions that might otherwise interfere with decision-making. Pain, fear, and uncertainty remain visible, but they are interpreted through a clinical lens rather than through personal identification.

This distance is not necessarily indifference. It is often a protective mechanism.

Medical professionals are exposed to suffering far more frequently than most people. If every encounter with illness were experienced with full emotional intensity, the psychological burden would become overwhelming. Detachment allows doctors to remain functional while performing difficult tasks.

Yet this protective adaptation can gradually reshape the doctor's relationship with patients.

The more the mind focuses on illness as a problem to solve, the easier it becomes to overlook the broader human experience surrounding that illness. Conversations become shorter and more structured. The doctor asks questions designed to identify symptoms rather than explore personal circumstances. Efficiency replaces narrative.

This change is rarely intentional. It emerges from the demands of clinical environments where time is limited and responsibility is high. The doctor must concentrate on solving medical problems, often within minutes.

But the psychological reshaping does not occur only in relation to patients. It also affects how doctors see themselves.

During the long journey of training, the individual gradually adopts the identity of a physician. Decision-making authority increases. The doctor becomes someone who must provide answers when others are uncertain. Patients and families begin to look toward the doctor for clarity and reassurance.

This authority carries both confidence and pressure.

Doctors must learn to speak with conviction even when medical outcomes remain uncertain. They must communicate complex information clearly while maintaining trust. They must accept that their decisions may influence the course of another person's life.

Living with such responsibility inevitably changes how a person thinks about risk, control, and accountability.

By the time a doctor completes training and begins practicing independently, the psychological reshaping is largely complete. The mind has adapted to operate within a world defined by clinical logic, rapid decision-making, and controlled emotional engagement.

The transformation has created a professional capable of navigating complex medical realities.

Yet it has also quietly introduced a tension that will follow the doctor throughout their career: the need to balance clinical objectivity with the human experience of illness.

This tension lies at the heart of modern medicine—and understanding it is essential to understanding what it truly means to become a doctor.

1.7 — The Birth of the Doctor

At the end of years of study, examinations, clinical postings, sleepless nights, and constant evaluation, a moment arrives that appears simple from the outside. A certificate is issued. A degree is awarded. The student who once sat in lecture halls is now officially called a doctor.

For many families, this moment carries deep pride. For the individual who has walked the long path of medical education, it feels like the completion of an enormous journey. The title "Doctor" suddenly becomes part of their identity.

Yet the birth of a doctor does not occur at the ceremony where the degree is handed over. It occurs gradually, through the accumulation of experiences that have quietly reshaped the person during the years of training.

By this stage, the young physician has already changed in ways that may not be immediately visible.

They have learned to think analytically in situations where others feel overwhelmed. They have developed the ability to observe symptoms and patterns quickly. They have practiced making decisions under pressure, sometimes with limited information and limited time. They have seen recovery, deterioration, and loss within the same hospital corridor.

These experiences create a professional who is capable of carrying responsibility that few other professions demand.

For the first time, the young doctor begins to operate with a certain degree of independence. Patients no longer see them only as students observing from the background. They see someone who can examine, diagnose, prescribe, and guide treatment. The doctor becomes a point of authority within the clinical environment.

This shift is significant.

Authority in medicine is not symbolic. It is functional. The advice given by a doctor can influence whether a patient undergoes surgery, begins medication, changes lifestyle habits, or prepares for long-term treatment. In many cases, medical decisions shape the course of another person's life.

With this authority comes a quiet realization: the profession is no longer about learning alone. It is about responsibility.

Every prescription carries potential consequences. Every clinical judgment affects real outcomes. Even routine consultations involve trust placed by patients who may not fully understand the complexity behind the doctor's decisions.

At the same time, the newly qualified doctor begins to recognize that knowledge itself is never complete. Medicine continues to evolve. New research, technologies, and treatments constantly reshape the field. The doctor who once felt relieved to have completed medical education soon discovers that learning must continue throughout their entire career.

Professional life therefore becomes an ongoing process of refinement rather than a finished achievement.

Another important realization also emerges during this phase. The young doctor enters a healthcare system that is far more complex than the academic environment in which they trained. Hospitals must balance patient care with administration, economics, infrastructure, and policy regulations. Doctors must navigate these systems while maintaining their clinical responsibilities.

The profession that once appeared straightforward now reveals multiple layers of complexity.

Within this environment, the doctor must learn to balance several roles simultaneously. They are a clinician responsible for diagnosis and treatment. They are a communicator who must explain difficult realities to patients and families. They are also a participant in a larger healthcare structure that influences how medicine is practiced.

These responsibilities define the real beginning of medical practice.

The birth of a doctor is therefore not simply the result of passing examinations or earning a degree. It is the emergence of a professional identity shaped by years of intellectual discipline, emotional adaptation, and practical experience.

Yet this transformation also raises an important question.

During the long journey of becoming a doctor, much has been gained—knowledge, authority, skill, and responsibility. But something may also have been quietly set aside along the way.

The curiosity that once asked *"Who is this person suffering?"* gradually evolves into the clinical question *"What disease is present?"*

Both questions are important. But when one begins to dominate the other, the relationship between doctor and patient begins to change.

Understanding this shift is essential to understanding modern medicine. Because the making of a doctor does not only create a healer—it also creates the mindset that will shape how patients are seen, understood, and treated in the years to come.

What Was Gained, What Was Left Behind

By the time the long journey of medical training reaches its end, the transformation is undeniable. The student who once entered medical school with curiosity and ambition has evolved into a professional equipped with extraordinary knowledge and responsibility. Years of study, discipline, and exposure to real clinical environments have shaped a mind capable of navigating complex medical realities.

Much has been gained in this process.

A doctor learns to observe the human body with precision. Symptoms that once seemed confusing now reveal patterns. Clinical reasoning develops into a powerful tool that allows physicians to move from uncertainty toward diagnosis and treatment. Knowledge that once existed only in textbooks becomes practical judgment in hospital wards and consultation rooms.

Equally important, the doctor develops resilience. Few professions demand the ability to function calmly in the presence of suffering, fear, and urgency. Through repeated exposure to difficult situations, doctors learn to remain steady when others around them may feel overwhelmed. This steadiness becomes one of the profession's most valuable strengths.

The journey also builds discipline and responsibility. A physician cannot approach decisions casually. Every prescription, every investigation, every intervention carries consequences. Medical training teaches doctors to think carefully, act methodically, and accept accountability for their judgments.

These qualities form the foundation of competent medical practice.

Yet the same journey that builds such strength also introduces subtle changes that often remain unnoticed. During the years of intense training, the doctor gradually learns to interpret human illness through structured frameworks. This is necessary for clinical efficiency, but it also shifts attention toward disease rather than experience.

Patients become identified through their conditions. A conversation begins with symptoms rather than stories. The doctor's mind moves quickly toward diagnosis, treatment plans, and measurable outcomes.

This shift does not happen because doctors lose compassion. It happens because medicine demands clarity and speed in environments where time is limited and decisions matter.

But in the process of sharpening clinical thinking, something delicate can slowly fade into the background—the full presence of the person who carries the illness.

The patient becomes easier to understand as a medical case than as a complex human being. The doctor becomes more comfortable analyzing pathology than engaging with the emotional realities that surround disease.

This change is rarely intentional. It is an adaptation to the pressures of medical practice. Yet over time, it shapes the nature of the doctor–patient relationship.

The profession gains extraordinary technical capability. At the same time, the human connection that once defined healing becomes more fragile.

Recognizing this tension is not a criticism of medicine. It is an invitation to understand the profession more honestly. Doctors do not operate in ideal conditions. They work within systems that demand efficiency, precision, and constant performance. The balance between science and humanity is therefore never simple.

But awareness of this balance matters.

Because the making of a doctor does not end with acquiring knowledge or mastering clinical procedures. It also involves continuously remembering that medicine exists not only to treat disease but to serve people who arrive with vulnerability, uncertainty, and trust.

The journey to becoming a doctor has created someone capable of extraordinary responsibility. The question that remains is how that responsibility will be carried.

The next chapter begins where this reflection leaves us—with a deeper look at what happens when the patient, slowly and almost invisibly, becomes something else.

A case.

Chapter 2 — When Humans Become Cases

The Language of the Ward

Walk through the corridor of any busy hospital ward and listen carefully to the conversations between doctors, nurses, and trainees. The language used inside these spaces is precise, efficient, and often very different from the way people speak about illness outside the hospital.

A patient lying in bed is rarely introduced by their name during clinical discussions. Instead, the patient becomes identified through their condition.

"The pneumonia in bed twelve needs review." "The diabetic case in the corner room is not responding to treatment." "Shift the fracture case for imaging."

To an outsider, this language may sound impersonal, even unsettling. It appears as though the individual has been replaced by the disease they carry. The person becomes secondary to the condition.

Yet within the hospital environment, this language is rarely intended to diminish the patient's humanity. It is a form of professional shorthand developed for clarity and speed. Hospitals are complex systems where dozens of patients require attention simultaneously. Doctors must communicate quickly, often while making critical decisions.

Referring to patients through their medical conditions allows teams to coordinate efficiently. The focus remains on diagnosis, treatment, and monitoring. In such settings, clinical language becomes a tool for organization rather than an expression of disregard.

However, language does more than transmit information. It shapes perception.

Over time, the repeated use of medical shorthand begins to influence how doctors think about patients. Instead of encountering a person with a unique life story, the physician increasingly encounters a set of symptoms belonging to a recognizable clinical pattern.

A middle-aged man experiencing stress, family responsibilities, and exhaustion gradually becomes a case of hypertension. A young woman dealing with fear and uncertainty becomes a surgical case awaiting intervention. An elderly patient who has lived through decades of experience becomes a geriatric complication risk.

None of these descriptions are medically incorrect. In fact, they are essential for diagnosis and treatment. But something subtle happens when the language of medicine becomes the primary lens through which patients are viewed.

The person carrying the illness slowly fades behind the illness itself.

This shift does not occur suddenly. It develops gradually as medical training encourages structured thinking. Students learn to identify patterns, isolate symptoms, and classify diseases. Clinical reasoning demands abstraction. Without it, the complexity of human illness would overwhelm even the most capable physician.

But the efficiency of abstraction carries a quiet consequence.

When humans are consistently discussed as cases, the doctor's attention naturally gravitates toward the disease rather than the individual. The consultation becomes centered on solving a biological problem. The patient's broader experience—fear, family pressures, financial concerns, personal identity—moves to the periphery.

In the fast-moving environment of modern healthcare, this transformation often goes unnoticed. Doctors are not consciously choosing to see people as cases. They are adapting to a system that rewards efficiency, accuracy, and speed.

Yet patients sense the difference immediately.

For them, the hospital visit is not a routine event. It is often a moment of vulnerability. They arrive carrying questions, anxieties, and hopes that extend far beyond the diagnosis written in their medical file. When the interaction feels rushed or narrowly focused on symptoms, patients may feel that something essential has been overlooked.

This difference in perception creates an invisible distance between doctor and patient.

On one side stands a professional trained to interpret illness through clinical frameworks. On the other stands a human being seeking not only treatment but recognition.

Understanding how this distance develops is essential to understanding modern medicine. Because the moment a human being becomes primarily a medical case marks a subtle turning point in the relationship between doctor and patient.

And that turning point rarely announces itself. It simply becomes part of the everyday language of the ward.

2.1 — Why Medicine Needs Categories

At first glance, the idea of reducing a human being to a medical category may seem uncomfortable. It can appear as though medicine strips away individuality in favor of technical labels. Yet this process did not emerge from indifference. It arose from necessity.

The human body is extraordinarily complex. Thousands of physiological processes occur simultaneously within it, each interacting with others in ways that are not always visible or predictable. When something goes wrong, the resulting symptoms can appear confusing, overlapping, and sometimes misleading. Without a structured way to organize these signals, diagnosing illness would become nearly impossible.

This is where medical categorization becomes essential.

Medicine developed classification systems to make sense of the enormous variety of diseases that affect the human body. Symptoms are grouped into recognizable patterns. Conditions are defined according to shared characteristics. Diagnostic frameworks allow doctors to narrow down possibilities and move toward effective treatment.

For example, a patient presenting with fever, cough, and breathing difficulty could be experiencing a wide range of conditions—from a mild infection to a serious respiratory disorder. By placing symptoms within known categories, doctors can evaluate probabilities, order appropriate tests, and begin treatment with greater precision.

In this way, categorization functions as a map. It helps doctors navigate the complex landscape of human illness.

Medical education therefore places strong emphasis on learning these categories. Students spend years studying disease classifications, diagnostic criteria, and treatment protocols. They are trained to recognize patterns quickly and accurately. A cluster of symptoms must immediately trigger a list of possible diagnoses. Each diagnosis must guide a logical sequence of investigations and interventions.

This approach transforms the overwhelming complexity of medicine into something manageable.

Clinical reasoning depends heavily on pattern recognition. Experienced doctors often identify probable conditions within minutes because they have encountered similar patterns many times before. What appears intuitive from the outside is actually the result of structured knowledge built through training and practice.

Categories also allow doctors to communicate efficiently with one another. When a physician describes a patient as having a particular condition, other professionals immediately understand the general nature of the problem, possible complications, and likely treatment strategies. This shared language ensures that medical teams can coordinate care effectively.

Without such organization, modern healthcare systems could not function.

Hospitals manage hundreds of patients simultaneously. Doctors, nurses, technicians, and specialists must work together within tight timeframes. Clear categories allow this collaboration to occur without confusion. Each professional understands the framework within which the patient's condition is being addressed.

Yet categorization has its limits.

Diseases may be classified neatly in textbooks, but real patients rarely fit perfectly into predefined boxes. Symptoms can overlap. Individuals may have multiple conditions simultaneously. Personal factors—such as stress, lifestyle, social environment, and emotional health—often influence how illness appears and progresses.

Despite these complexities, the medical mind must begin somewhere. Categories provide the starting point for understanding.

They allow doctors to approach illness systematically rather than randomly. They reduce uncertainty and create pathways toward treatment. Without them, medicine would lose the clarity that makes diagnosis and intervention possible.

However, while categories are powerful tools for managing disease, they do not capture the full reality of the person experiencing that disease.

A diagnosis may describe what is happening inside the body, but it cannot fully represent the human life that surrounds that condition. The patient remains more complex than any classification.

Understanding this difference is crucial. Because the same categories that make medicine effective can also quietly narrow the lens through which doctors view those who come to them for help.

The challenge for modern medicine is therefore not to abandon categories—they are indispensable—but to remember that they are tools, not definitions of the person who carries the illness.

2.2 — From Story to Symptoms

When a patient first enters a hospital or clinic, they rarely begin by describing their illness in clinical terms. They arrive with a story.

They speak about how the problem began, what they were doing at the time, how it has affected their daily life, and how worried they feel about what might happen next. The story may include family concerns, financial pressure, interrupted work, or sleepless nights spent thinking about the illness. For the patient, the disease is not a collection of symptoms; it is an event that has disrupted the rhythm of life.

The doctor, however, must listen to this story with a different objective.

Medical training teaches physicians to translate narratives into medically useful information. During a consultation, the doctor carefully guides the conversation toward specific details: when the symptoms started, how severe they are, what makes them better or worse, whether similar problems have occurred before, and what other conditions might be present.

This process is known as history taking, and it is one of the most important tools in medicine.

Through a structured set of questions, the doctor gradually transforms a complex human narrative into clinical data that can be analyzed. Personal descriptions become measurable observations.

Vague discomfort becomes localized pain. Emotional concerns are filtered to reveal physical symptoms.

For example, a patient might begin by saying, "I haven't been feeling well for weeks. I feel tired all the time, and I'm worried something is seriously wrong."

The doctor must gently redirect this statement into precise medical information:

How long has the fatigue been present? Is it constant or intermittent? Is it associated with fever, weight loss, or shortness of breath? Are there any other symptoms?

Each question narrows the field of possibilities. Gradually, the patient's story is distilled into a clinical pattern that the doctor can evaluate.

This translation from story to symptoms is not meant to ignore the patient's experience. It is designed to identify the underlying cause of illness as accurately as possible. Without focusing on specific details, diagnosis would become unreliable.

Yet something important happens during this process.

The richness of the patient's narrative often becomes compressed into a few medically relevant points. A long personal story may be summarized in a short clinical note. The emotional dimension of the illness may be acknowledged but not explored in depth, especially in busy clinical settings where time is limited.

The doctor's attention moves toward identifying the biological disturbance that must be treated.

From the physician's perspective, this narrowing of focus is necessary. A doctor may see dozens of patients in a single day. Each consultation must gather essential information efficiently so that appropriate investigations and treatments can begin. Without this structured approach, the healthcare system would struggle to function.

But from the patient's perspective, the experience can feel very different.

A person who arrives hoping to share their concerns fully may feel that the conversation has been redirected too quickly toward symptoms and tests. The patient may leave the consultation with treatment instructions but with the feeling that their broader experience was only partially understood.

This difference in perspective highlights a central tension within medical practice.

Doctors are trained to interpret illness scientifically. Patients experience illness personally. One seeks patterns and causes; the other seeks understanding and reassurance.

The translation from story to symptoms therefore represents one of the most important—and most delicate—moments in the doctor–patient relationship.

If done carefully, it allows doctors to gather the information necessary for accurate diagnosis while still acknowledging the person behind the illness. If done too mechanically, it can unintentionally reduce a complex human experience into a narrow clinical summary.

Over time, repeated consultations strengthen the doctor's ability to extract symptoms quickly and efficiently. The skill becomes almost automatic. The physician learns to identify the medically relevant pieces of information within moments of hearing the patient's narrative.

This efficiency is valuable in clinical practice.

But it also marks another step in the transformation explored in this chapter: the gradual movement from engaging with a human story to analyzing a medical case.

2.3 — The Efficiency of Abstraction

Hospitals are environments where time moves differently from the outside world. A doctor working in a busy outpatient department may see dozens of patients in a single day. In emergency wards and intensive care units, the pace can be even more intense. Every patient requires attention, yet time remains limited. Decisions must often be made quickly and with clarity.

In such conditions, medicine cannot rely on long, open-ended conversations or slow reflection. It requires a way to process complex information efficiently. This is where abstraction becomes one of the most important tools in clinical practice.

Abstraction allows doctors to simplify complicated realities without losing essential meaning. Instead of holding every detail of a patient's life in mind, the physician focuses on the elements that are most relevant to diagnosis and treatment. Symptoms are grouped together, patterns are recognized, and the situation is translated into a manageable medical framework.

For example, a patient might describe weeks of fatigue, stress at work, irregular sleep, poor appetite, and occasional headaches. All of these experiences are real and important within the patient's life. However, the doctor must determine whether these symptoms point toward a specific medical condition. To do this, the physician isolates key indicators, evaluates possible causes, and organizes the information within known clinical categories.

This process turns a complex life situation into a medical problem that can be addressed through investigation and treatment.

Abstraction therefore functions as a form of mental compression. It reduces overwhelming complexity into something that can be analyzed logically. Without this ability, doctors would struggle to manage the sheer volume of information they encounter each day.

Clinical shorthand is one of the visible results of this process. Doctors communicate with each other using concise descriptions that immediately convey essential details. A phrase such as "a diabetic patient with uncontrolled blood sugar" quickly signals a set of risks, possible complications, and treatment considerations. Within seconds, another doctor understands the general situation.

This efficiency is vital in environments where delays can affect outcomes.

Emergency medicine provides a clear example. When a critically ill patient arrives, the medical team cannot spend long periods discussing personal narratives. The focus must immediately shift to stabilizing the patient. Vital signs are assessed, symptoms are interpreted, and treatment begins rapidly. In such moments, abstraction allows doctors to move from observation to action without hesitation.

Yet the efficiency of abstraction has consequences that extend beyond clinical decision-making.

When the mind repeatedly compresses human situations into medical categories, it becomes easier to see the illness rather than the individual carrying it. The doctor begins to interact with the disease as a problem to be solved rather than with the patient as a person navigating illness.

This shift is not the result of neglect or lack of compassion. It is a byproduct of the environment in which modern medicine operates. Doctors must function within systems that reward speed, accuracy, and productivity. Consultation times may be limited. Administrative responsibilities compete with patient interaction. Technological tools generate large amounts of data that require interpretation.

Under these pressures, abstraction becomes indispensable.

However, the more medicine relies on abstraction, the more carefully doctors must remain aware of its limits. While abstraction simplifies clinical reasoning, it cannot fully represent the human experience surrounding illness.

A diagnosis may describe the biological condition, but it does not capture the emotional and social dimensions of living with that condition. The medical category identifies the disease, but it does not describe the person.

Recognizing this difference becomes an important part of professional maturity. Doctors must use abstraction to manage complexity, yet they must also remember that every case represents a human life that extends beyond the boundaries of clinical categories.

This balance is not always easy to maintain, especially in environments where time and pressure push doctors toward efficiency.

But understanding the power—and the limitation—of abstraction is essential for anyone seeking to understand how humans slowly become cases within the modern practice of medicine.

2.4 — The Emotional Distance of Clinical Thinking

Medicine is one of the few professions where a person repeatedly encounters human vulnerability at its most intense moments. Patients arrive in pain, frightened by uncertainty, worried about their future, and often accompanied by families who carry their own fears. For a young medical student or trainee, these encounters can be emotionally overwhelming at first.

In the early stages of training, many students react with deep empathy. The suffering of patients feels personal. The distress of families lingers in the mind even after leaving the hospital. Witnessing serious illness or death can create strong emotional responses that are difficult to process.

However, clinical practice demands that doctors continue functioning regardless of these emotions.

A physician cannot allow fear, sadness, or anxiety to interfere with the ability to think clearly. Diagnosis requires concentration. Treatment requires careful decision-making. In emergency situations, hesitation caused by emotional overload can delay critical action.

For this reason, medical training gradually teaches doctors to develop a form of emotional distance.

This distance is not meant to eliminate compassion. Instead, it allows the doctor to remain stable while working in situations that would otherwise become psychologically exhausting. The physician learns to observe suffering without being overwhelmed by it, to acknowledge distress without becoming immobilized by it.

In practical terms, this emotional distance allows doctors to perform tasks that might otherwise be unbearable.

A surgeon must focus on the technical precision of an operation rather than the fear of the patient lying on the table. An emergency physician must move quickly from one critical case to another without carrying the emotional weight of each encounter into the next. A resident in an intensive care unit must make decisions even when the outcome remains uncertain.

Clinical thinking therefore encourages a mental framework that prioritizes clarity and control. The doctor analyzes symptoms, evaluates data, and determines treatment options with professional focus. Emotions remain present but are carefully regulated so they do not disrupt the decision-making process.

Over time, this adaptation becomes part of the doctor's professional identity.

What once required conscious effort gradually becomes instinctive. The physician learns to shift into a clinical mindset whenever a patient interaction begins. Questions are asked systematically, examinations follow established procedures, and treatment plans are developed with efficiency.

From the outside, this behavior can sometimes appear cold or impersonal.

Patients who are experiencing illness for the first time may expect a more openly emotional response from their doctor. When the physician maintains a calm, analytical tone, it can be misinterpreted as indifference. In reality, the doctor may simply be operating within the mental discipline that medical training has reinforced.

Yet emotional distance carries its own risks.

When clinical detachment becomes too strong, the doctor may begin to lose awareness of how illness feels from the patient's perspective. Conversations may become shorter and more technical. Emotional cues from patients may go unnoticed. The consultation may focus almost entirely on medical details.

At this point, the protective mechanism that once helped the doctor function effectively can begin to weaken the connection between doctor and patient.

The challenge lies in maintaining balance.

Too much emotional involvement can exhaust the doctor and interfere with professional judgment. Too much distance can make patients feel unseen and unheard. Effective medical practice requires a careful equilibrium between compassion and clinical clarity.

Achieving this balance is not easy. It evolves through experience, reflection, and sometimes through mistakes that teach the doctor to adjust their approach.

For many physicians, the process of learning how to remain both human and professional becomes one of the most difficult aspects of the profession.

Because the emotional distance that medicine requires is not simply a technique—it is part of the psychological transformation that occurs when a person becomes a doctor.

2.5 — The Patient's Experience

While clinical thinking organizes illness into categories and symptoms, the experience of being a patient unfolds in an entirely different way. For the person seeking medical help, illness rarely feels like a structured problem waiting to be solved. It feels like disruption.

A patient enters the hospital or clinic at a moment when something in life has gone wrong. The body is not functioning normally. There may be pain, weakness, or unexplained changes that create fear. Even when the symptoms appear minor, uncertainty can be unsettling. Many patients arrive not only for treatment but for reassurance that their lives will return to normal.

In that moment, the doctor represents knowledge, authority, and hope.

Patients look to the physician not simply for a prescription or test result but for understanding. They want someone to recognize the seriousness of what they are experiencing. They want their concerns to be heard and interpreted with care.

However, the clinical environment often moves faster than the patient expects.

Consultations may be brief. Questions focus quickly on specific symptoms. The doctor examines, reviews reports, and proposes a plan of treatment. From the physician's perspective, this efficiency reflects professional competence. From the patient's perspective, the interaction may feel incomplete.

Many patients leave the consultation with an uneasy feeling that their story was only partially understood.

This experience becomes even more pronounced in large hospitals where the number of patients is high. Waiting rooms fill with people who have already spent hours anticipating their appointment. When the actual conversation with the doctor lasts only a few minutes, the contrast between expectation and reality becomes noticeable.

The patient may wonder whether the doctor truly grasped the full picture of their situation.

In addition to physical symptoms, patients often carry emotional burdens into the consultation. Illness can disrupt work, family responsibilities, and financial stability. A person who suddenly becomes sick may worry about how treatment will affect their ability to support their family or maintain daily routines.

These concerns may not always appear in medical charts, but they strongly influence how patients experience their illness.

When the consultation focuses narrowly on clinical details, these broader worries may remain unspoken. Patients may hesitate to bring them up, sensing that the doctor is already pressed for time. As a result, the encounter becomes primarily technical.

For the patient, the illness remains deeply personal. For the doctor, it becomes part of a larger clinical workload.

This difference in perspective can gradually affect trust.

If patients feel that their individuality has been reduced to a medical condition, they may begin to question whether the healthcare system sees them as people or simply as cases to be processed. Even when the treatment itself is correct and effective, the experience of the consultation can influence how patients perceive their care.

It is important to recognize that this perception is rarely caused by a lack of dedication from doctors. Most physicians enter the profession with a sincere desire to help people. Yet the pressures of modern healthcare—large patient volumes, administrative demands, and time constraints—often limit how much attention can be given to each individual encounter.

The patient, however, measures the quality of care differently.

While doctors evaluate success through diagnosis and treatment outcomes, patients often evaluate their experience through communication and empathy. A patient who feels heard and understood may accept even difficult medical news with greater trust. A patient who feels overlooked may carry lingering dissatisfaction even when the medical care was technically correct.

Understanding the patient's experience is therefore essential to understanding the larger transformation described in this chapter.

Because the moment when a human being feels reduced to a medical case is not defined by clinical categories alone. It is defined by the absence of recognition—the feeling that the person behind the illness has disappeared from the conversation.

For medicine to function effectively, doctors must analyze symptoms and diagnose diseases. But for patients to feel truly cared for, they must remain visible as individuals within that process.

Bridging this difference between clinical reasoning and human experience remains one of the central challenges of modern medical practice.

2.6 — The Doctor's Dilemma

From the outside, the doctor–patient interaction often appears straightforward. A patient arrives with a problem, the doctor examines the condition, and treatment is provided. Yet behind this seemingly simple exchange lies a complex web of pressures that shape how medicine is practiced.

Doctors rarely operate in isolation. They work within systems that demand efficiency, accountability, and constant performance. Hospitals must manage large numbers of patients, maintain infrastructure, coordinate multiple departments, and comply with regulations and administrative procedures. Within this environment, the doctor becomes both a healer and a participant in a larger institutional structure.

This creates a dilemma that many physicians quietly experience but rarely articulate.

On one side lies the ideal image of medicine: a doctor listening patiently, understanding the patient's concerns, carefully examining the illness, and providing thoughtful guidance. On the other side lies the operational reality of modern healthcare: crowded clinics, limited consultation time, extensive documentation, and pressure to manage a high volume of cases.

A doctor working in a busy outpatient department may need to see dozens of patients in a single day. Each patient expects attention and reassurance. At the same time, hospital administrators monitor efficiency, waiting times, and service capacity. Delays create dissatisfaction not only among patients but also within the system that must keep functioning.

In such circumstances, the doctor must constantly balance competing priorities.

Spending more time with one patient means less time available for others waiting outside. A detailed conversation may provide comfort to a worried individual, but it may also slow the pace of the clinic and extend waiting times for everyone else.

These decisions are rarely simple.

In addition to patient interactions, doctors face growing administrative responsibilities. Medical records must be maintained carefully. Reports must be written. Legal documentation must be completed accurately. Communication with insurance providers, hospital management, and regulatory bodies often requires additional time and attention.

All of these tasks compete with the time available for direct patient care.

Technology has also introduced new complexities. While diagnostic tools and digital systems have improved medical accuracy, they have also created environments where doctors spend significant time reviewing screens, reports, and electronic records. In many consultations, the physician's attention must move repeatedly between the patient and the data generated by machines.

This dynamic can unintentionally shift the center of interaction away from the person and toward the information surrounding them.

Within these pressures, doctors must still maintain clinical accuracy and professional judgment. Every decision must be defensible, both medically and legally. The fear of making an error—particularly in an era of increasing scrutiny and litigation—adds another layer of stress to everyday practice.

Under such conditions, the doctor often turns toward structured clinical thinking as a way to maintain control.

By focusing on symptoms, diagnoses, and treatment protocols, physicians can navigate complexity more efficiently. The patient's condition becomes part of a recognizable medical framework that guides decision-making. This approach reduces uncertainty and helps the doctor manage large workloads without losing clinical clarity.

However, the same strategy that protects the doctor from chaos can unintentionally distance them from the human experience of illness.

Doctors themselves are often aware of this tension. Many recognize that patients need more than clinical answers—they need reassurance, explanation, and understanding. Yet the system within which medicine operates does not always allow these needs to be addressed fully.

This is the heart of the doctor's dilemma.

The physician must treat patients with care while functioning within structures that demand speed and efficiency. They must balance empathy with practicality, listening with time constraints, and personal attention with institutional responsibility.

It is easy for observers to interpret short consultations or clinical language as signs of indifference. But for many doctors, these behaviors are adaptations to the realities of modern healthcare rather than reflections of personal values.

Recognizing this dilemma does not excuse shortcomings in communication or compassion. Instead, it helps explain why the transformation from human stories to medical cases occurs so easily within contemporary medicine.

Because the doctor is not only responding to individual patients. The doctor is also responding to the system that surrounds every consultation.

Understanding this tension is essential if the relationship between doctors and patients is to remain meaningful in an increasingly complex healthcare world.

2.7 — Recovering the Human Without Losing the Science

If clinical thinking inevitably transforms human stories into medical cases, the question that follows is unavoidable: can medicine retain its scientific clarity while still preserving the human dimension of care?

This question does not challenge the foundations of modern medicine. Scientific discipline is what allows doctors to diagnose accurately, treat effectively, and save lives. Without structured knowledge, clinical reasoning, and evidence-based practice, healthcare would quickly descend into uncertainty and inconsistency.

Science must therefore remain the backbone of medical practice.

Yet the presence of science does not require the disappearance of the human being behind the illness. The real challenge lies in ensuring that scientific thinking does not become so dominant that it overshadows the person who carries the disease.

Recovering this balance begins with recognizing a simple truth: illness never exists only inside the body.

Every patient arrives with a life that continues beyond the hospital walls. A diagnosis affects not only biological systems but also emotional stability, family relationships, financial security, and personal identity. For some patients, the illness itself may be less frightening than the uncertainty it introduces into their future.

Doctors cannot resolve all of these concerns through medical treatment alone. However, awareness of these dimensions can significantly influence how care is delivered.

Sometimes the difference lies not in the treatment plan but in the way it is communicated.

A patient who understands the nature of their condition and feels that their concerns have been acknowledged is more likely to trust the medical process. Even brief conversations that allow patients to ask questions and receive clear explanations can restore a sense of partnership between doctor and patient.

Communication, therefore, becomes an essential clinical skill rather than an optional courtesy.

A physician who can explain complex medical situations in clear and respectful language helps patients navigate uncertainty with greater confidence. In many cases, reassurance emerges not from promising perfect outcomes but from demonstrating thoughtful attention to the patient's situation.

Recovering the human dimension of medicine also requires a shift in how doctors perceive their role.

Instead of seeing themselves only as problem-solvers addressing biological disturbances, doctors can recognize that they occupy a unique position within moments of vulnerability in human life. Patients approach them not only for technical expertise but also for guidance through situations they do not fully understand.

This recognition does not require dramatic changes in medical practice. Often it involves small adjustments in awareness.

A doctor who briefly acknowledges a patient's worry before discussing test results, who pauses long enough to allow a question, or who explains the reasoning behind a treatment decision can transform the tone of a consultation. Such moments remind patients that they are not simply cases within a system but individuals receiving care.

Importantly, restoring this balance does not mean slowing medicine to an impractical pace. Modern healthcare systems will continue to operate under constraints of time and resources. Efficiency will remain necessary.

What can change is the awareness with which efficiency is applied.

Clinical categories and diagnostic frameworks will always remain essential tools. They allow doctors to manage complexity and deliver effective treatment. But when these tools are recognized as instruments rather than definitions of the patient, the physician's perspective widens again.

The case becomes a person carrying a condition.

Science continues to guide diagnosis and treatment, but humanity remains present in the interaction.

For many experienced doctors, this balance emerges naturally with time. Years of practice teach that medicine is not only about solving clinical puzzles but about participating in moments where knowledge, uncertainty, and trust intersect.

In such moments, the doctor's role extends beyond technical expertise. It becomes a form of stewardship—guiding patients through illness with both scientific competence and human awareness.

Recovering the human without losing the science is therefore not a rejection of modern medicine. It is an evolution of it.

And recognizing this possibility brings the chapter back to its central theme: understanding how humans become cases is the first step toward ensuring that cases never completely replace the humans they represent.

The Case and the Person

Medicine cannot function without cases. Every day in hospitals and clinics, doctors must identify diseases, classify symptoms, and organize information into patterns that can be understood and treated. Without this structure, the practice of medicine would lose its clarity and reliability.

Clinical categories therefore serve an essential purpose. They allow physicians to navigate complexity, communicate with colleagues, and make decisions with precision. In many situations, this structured thinking saves lives.

Yet within this efficiency lies a quiet paradox.

The very process that allows doctors to treat disease effectively can also obscure the person who carries that disease. The patient who entered the hospital as a human being with a life, relationships, responsibilities, and fears gradually becomes represented by a diagnosis.

A case file replaces a conversation. A medical chart summarizes a personal struggle. A condition becomes the central identity of the patient within the clinical environment.

This transformation is rarely intentional. It emerges naturally from the demands of medical practice. Doctors must process large amounts of information quickly. They must prioritize biological signals that indicate danger or recovery. In such circumstances, abstraction becomes a practical necessity.

But when abstraction becomes the dominant lens through which patients are seen, something important is lost.

Illness does not occur in isolation from life. A diagnosis interacts with the patient's world—family members waiting anxiously for updates, careers interrupted by treatment, financial pressures that influence decisions, and emotional responses that shape how individuals cope with uncertainty.

These realities may not appear in laboratory reports, yet they strongly influence how patients experience illness and recovery.

For doctors, recognizing this broader human context does not mean abandoning clinical discipline. It simply means remembering that every medical category points toward a person whose life extends far beyond the boundaries of a hospital bed.

The physician must therefore learn to hold two perspectives simultaneously.

One perspective focuses on disease: identifying patterns, analyzing symptoms, and determining treatment. This is the scientific core of medicine, and it must remain rigorous.

The other perspective focuses on the human being who carries the illness: a person navigating fear, hope, responsibility, and uncertainty. This dimension cannot always be solved with medical intervention, but it can be acknowledged through awareness and communication.

When these two perspectives remain balanced, the doctor–patient relationship retains its depth.

The case becomes a tool for understanding the illness. The person remains the reason the illness matters.

Maintaining this balance is not always easy. The pressures of modern healthcare systems constantly push medicine toward efficiency and abstraction. Time constraints, administrative responsibilities, and institutional demands encourage doctors to focus on measurable outcomes.

Yet within these pressures, the awareness that every case represents a human life can quietly shape how medicine is practiced.

A brief explanation offered to a worried patient, a moment taken to listen before prescribing treatment, or a thoughtful response to a family member's concern can restore the sense that the patient remains visible within the system.

These gestures may seem small, but they carry profound meaning for those experiencing illness.

Because at the heart of medicine lies a simple truth: diseases may be categorized, analyzed, and treated, but healing always involves people.

Recognizing this difference does not weaken medical science. It strengthens the purpose behind it.

The next chapter explores another dimension of this transformation—the emotional distance that doctors develop in order to survive the demands of their profession, and the cost that this distance can quietly impose on both the physician and the patient.

Chapter 3 — The Emotional Cost of Detachment

The Moment the Heart Steps Back

In the early days of medical training, many students encounter illness with a natural emotional response. The first time they stand beside a patient in pain, watch a family waiting anxiously outside a ward, or witness the fragile condition of someone fighting for life, the experience leaves a deep impression. For a young trainee, the hospital is not just a place of learning—it is a place where human vulnerability becomes visible in its most direct form.

During these moments, the instinctive reaction is empathy. The suffering of the patient feels immediate and personal. Students may carry these experiences in their minds long after leaving the hospital corridors. A difficult case, a grieving family, or the quiet stillness that follows an unsuccessful resuscitation can linger in memory for days.

At the beginning of this journey, the student often believes that feeling deeply is part of what will make them a good doctor.

Yet as training progresses, the reality of medical practice begins to change that expectation.

Hospitals do not present suffering as a rare event. They present it repeatedly, day after day. Patients arrive continuously with illness, injury, fear, and uncertainty. Some recover quickly. Others remain in critical condition. A few do not survive despite every effort made by the medical team.

For a doctor responsible for treating many patients, responding to each situation with full emotional intensity becomes difficult to sustain.

Gradually, something subtle begins to happen. The mind learns to step back—not out of cruelty or indifference, but out of necessity. The doctor discovers that if every case is experienced with the same emotional depth as the first, the weight of the profession becomes impossible to carry.

So the heart takes a small step backward.

This step is not immediately visible, even to the doctor themselves. It appears in small ways: focusing more on clinical details than emotional reactions, moving quickly from one patient to the next, maintaining a calm tone even in situations where families are distressed.

From the outside, this behavior may look like emotional distance. From the doctor's perspective, it is often the only way to remain steady in a profession filled with unpredictable outcomes.

Clinical practice demands clarity of thought. A physician facing a critical situation cannot allow panic or grief to interfere with judgment. Decisions must be made quickly and carefully. Treatment must continue even when emotions run high.

The ability to regulate emotional responses therefore becomes part of professional discipline.

Yet the moment when the heart steps back marks an important transition in the life of a doctor. It is the beginning of a protective mechanism that allows physicians to continue practicing medicine despite constant exposure to human suffering.

This adaptation helps doctors function effectively, but it also introduces a delicate balance. The same emotional distance that protects the physician can, over time, reshape how patients are perceived and how interactions unfold.

Understanding this moment—the quiet step back of the heart—is essential to understanding the emotional cost that medicine sometimes carries, both for doctors and for those who seek their care.

3.1 — The First Shock of Human Suffering

Before entering medical training, most students encounter illness only occasionally. A family member may fall sick, a neighbor may be hospitalized, or a news story may mention a medical emergency. These events are serious, but they remain distant from everyday life. For many young students, suffering appears as something rare—an interruption in normal living rather than a constant presence.

Medical education changes that perception quickly.

When students begin their clinical postings, they are suddenly placed in environments where illness is not an exception but the central reality. Wards are filled with patients experiencing pain, weakness, anxiety, and uncertainty. Emergency rooms receive people whose lives have been abruptly disrupted by accidents, infections, heart attacks, and countless other conditions.

For the first time, the student stands directly inside the world of human suffering.

These early encounters often carry a strong emotional impact. A medical student may feel nervous when approaching a patient for the first time, unsure of how to ask questions or conduct an examination while someone is clearly uncomfortable. The awareness that another human being is depending on the medical team for relief creates a sense of responsibility that can feel overwhelming.

In the beginning, the student's emotional response is often intense.

Watching a patient struggle to breathe, hearing a family member speak with fear in their voice, or observing the quiet tension that surrounds a critically ill person can leave lasting impressions. Some students find themselves thinking about these situations long after they leave the hospital for the day.

Among the most powerful experiences during this period is witnessing the limits of medicine.

In textbooks, treatments are presented with clear outcomes and logical progressions. In real clinical environments, outcomes are not always predictable. A patient who seemed stable may deteriorate suddenly. A treatment that works for one individual may fail for another. Despite the best efforts of the medical team, there are moments when recovery does not occur.

For a young trainee encountering such situations for the first time, the realization can be deeply unsettling.

Students who entered medical school with the hope of helping people quickly discover that medicine involves confronting the boundaries of human capability. Not every illness can be reversed. Not every life can be saved.

These experiences create the first emotional shock of clinical training.

Some students respond by becoming more determined to learn and improve their skills. Others struggle with the emotional weight of what they witness. Conversations with peers often reveal that many trainees feel uncertain about how to process these moments.

At this stage, the student is still experiencing illness primarily through empathy.

They imagine themselves or their family members in the patient's situation. The suffering feels personal, even though the student is not directly responsible for the outcome. The emotional intensity of these early encounters can make the hospital environment feel overwhelming.

Yet the clinical environment continues moving forward regardless of individual feelings.

New patients arrive. New cases must be examined. The daily rhythm of the hospital does not pause to allow extended reflection. Students gradually learn that the profession requires them to remain present and functional even when situations evoke strong emotions.

This realization marks the beginning of a significant psychological adjustment.

The student begins to understand that medicine demands more than knowledge and technical skill. It requires the ability to face suffering repeatedly without losing the capacity to act effectively.

The first shock of human suffering therefore becomes an early lesson in the emotional realities of medical practice. It introduces the future doctor to a world where compassion must coexist with composure, and where the human response to pain must gradually be shaped into professional resilience.

3.2 — Learning to Control Emotion

After the first encounters with suffering, young medical trainees quickly realize that emotional response alone cannot guide clinical practice. Compassion may motivate the desire to help, but it does not provide the clarity required to diagnose illness, make treatment decisions, or manage critical situations.

Medicine demands something more disciplined: the ability to regulate emotion while continuing to think clearly.

During the early years of clinical exposure, students begin to observe how experienced doctors behave in difficult situations. A senior physician may deliver serious news to a patient with calm composure. A surgeon may remain completely focused during a complicated procedure while the atmosphere in the operating room becomes tense. An emergency doctor may move swiftly from one critically ill patient to another without visible hesitation.

For students watching these interactions, the behavior of senior doctors can appear almost detached. The calmness seems unusual in situations where emotions might easily overwhelm others. Yet this composure is not a lack of feeling. It is the result of deliberate professional discipline.

Doctors learn that emotions must be acknowledged but carefully managed.

If a physician allows fear or distress to dominate the mind during a medical emergency, decision-making becomes impaired. Treatment requires attention to details—vital signs, medication dosages, laboratory values, procedural steps. These tasks demand concentration, and concentration requires emotional control.

Medical training therefore gradually encourages the development of this control.

Students learn to shift their focus from emotional reaction to clinical observation. When confronted with a difficult case, they are guided to ask structured questions: What are the symptoms? What are the possible diagnoses? What investigations are needed? What treatment should begin immediately?

This approach helps transform overwhelming situations into manageable clinical problems.

Over time, trainees begin practicing this discipline themselves. The first time they encounter a patient in severe distress, their instinct may be to react emotionally. But as training continues, they learn to pause, assess the situation systematically, and respond with professional clarity.

The goal is not to eliminate empathy but to prevent emotional paralysis.

There is an important difference between empathy and emotional immersion. Empathy allows a doctor to recognize the patient's experience and respond with concern. Emotional immersion, however, can make it difficult to maintain the objectivity required for effective treatment.

A doctor who becomes completely absorbed in a patient's distress may struggle to make rational decisions. The profession therefore encourages a form of empathy that remains balanced with clinical reasoning.

This process is reinforced repeatedly throughout training. Clinical discussions focus on symptoms, diagnostic pathways, and treatment plans rather than emotional responses. Case presentations emphasize facts and medical interpretation. Even when situations are emotionally difficult, the language of medicine remains analytical.

Gradually, this approach shapes the doctor's internal habits.

The physician learns to enter what might be called a *clinical mindset*—a mental state where observation, analysis, and decision-making take priority over emotional reaction. This mindset allows doctors to function effectively in environments where suffering is common and time-sensitive decisions are required.

However, learning to control emotion also introduces subtle changes in how doctors relate to patients.

The more frequently physicians rely on clinical discipline, the more natural emotional restraint becomes. Conversations may become more focused on symptoms and treatment rather than personal experience. The doctor's attention shifts toward solving medical problems rather than exploring emotional contexts.

This change is rarely intentional. It simply reflects the professional training that enables doctors to remain effective under pressure.

Yet the ability to control emotion—so necessary for medical practice—also marks another step in the transformation of the physician. The heart that once responded instinctively to suffering learns to step aside long enough for the mind to act with precision.

This discipline protects both doctor and patient.

But it also carries a question that will continue to echo throughout the profession: how much emotional distance is necessary, and at what point does control begin to resemble detachment?

3.3 — Repetition and Desensitization

One of the most powerful forces shaping a doctor's emotional world is not a single dramatic event but repetition. In the early stages of training, every encounter with illness feels intense and memorable. The student notices the expressions on patients' faces, the anxiety of family members, the tension in hospital corridors, and the seriousness of medical conversations.

But hospitals are environments where such moments occur constantly.

Day after day, doctors see patients struggling with pain, fear, and uncertainty. New admissions arrive continuously. Emergency cases interrupt routines. Serious diagnoses are discussed. Surgical procedures take place. Recoveries occur, but so do complications.

What initially feels extraordinary gradually becomes familiar.

This familiarity is not the result of indifference. It is the natural psychological response to repeated exposure. The human mind adapts to experiences that occur frequently. What once appeared overwhelming slowly becomes part of the normal rhythm of daily work.

For doctors, this process of adaptation often begins during residency.

A resident may spend long hours in wards where critically ill patients require constant monitoring. They may witness numerous medical emergencies within a short period. The urgency that once created strong emotional reactions slowly becomes part of the expected environment.

In such settings, emotional responses begin to soften.

A young trainee who once felt deeply shaken by a difficult case may now respond with professional composure. The mind focuses more on clinical tasks than on emotional interpretation. The doctor learns to observe suffering without reacting to it with the same intensity as before.

This psychological adjustment is often referred to as desensitization.

Desensitization allows doctors to function effectively in environments where emotional overload would otherwise become debilitating. If every difficult case triggered the same emotional shock as the first encounter, doctors would struggle to maintain the concentration required for clinical work.

Instead, the mind gradually learns to treat these experiences as part of professional life.

For example, a medical student might initially feel distressed while observing a patient in severe pain. After years of training, the same situation prompts a different response. The doctor quickly evaluates the symptoms, determines the cause, and begins treatment without pausing for emotional reaction.

The suffering has not become less real, but the doctor's response has changed.

This transformation can be seen in the language doctors use among themselves. Conversations often focus on clinical details rather than emotional aspects. A difficult situation may be described through diagnostic terms or procedural steps rather than through expressions of personal distress.

Such language reflects the professional mindset that develops through repeated exposure.

However, desensitization carries both benefits and risks.

On the positive side, it strengthens the doctor's ability to remain calm under pressure. Physicians who have encountered many challenging situations often develop remarkable composure. They can approach critical moments with clarity and confidence, which benefits patients who depend on their stability.

But desensitization can also gradually narrow the emotional lens through which doctors see their work.

When suffering becomes routine, it may no longer evoke the same level of reflection it once did. The doctor becomes accustomed to situations that patients and families experience as extraordinary. What feels normal within the hospital may still feel devastating for those encountering illness for the first time.

This difference in perspective can quietly influence the doctor–patient relationship.

A physician who has witnessed countless medical cases may unconsciously respond with efficiency rather than emotional acknowledgment. The doctor moves quickly toward diagnosis and treatment, while the patient is still processing the shock of illness.

Neither perspective is wrong. They simply emerge from different experiences of the same situation.

For doctors, desensitization is part of learning how to survive the demands of medical practice. It allows them to continue functioning in environments where emotional intensity is unavoidable.

Yet it also reminds us that professional adaptation always carries a human cost. The repeated exposure that strengthens clinical resilience may simultaneously create distance between the doctor's professional routine and the patient's deeply personal experience of illness.

3.4 — The Protective Shield of Detachment

As medical training progresses and exposure to suffering becomes routine, doctors begin to develop a psychological shield. This shield is not taught formally in classrooms, nor is it written in textbooks. It emerges gradually through experience as physicians learn how to protect themselves from the emotional weight of the profession.

This shield is detachment.

Detachment allows doctors to remain functional in situations that would otherwise become emotionally overwhelming. When a physician faces patients who are critically ill, grieving families, or uncertain outcomes, the ability to step back emotionally becomes a form of self-preservation. Without this boundary, the emotional impact of the profession could quickly accumulate beyond what any individual could bear.

In practical terms, detachment helps doctors maintain clarity in moments where others may feel panic or distress.

A surgeon entering an operating room cannot focus on the anxiety of the patient or the tension of the family waiting outside. The surgeon must concentrate on anatomy, precision, and technique. An emergency physician responding to a cardiac arrest must focus entirely on the sequence of life-saving interventions. Emotional reaction must wait until after the immediate crisis has passed.

Detachment therefore becomes a functional skill.

It allows doctors to perform tasks that require intense concentration while remaining unaffected by emotional turbulence around them. In environments such as intensive care units, trauma centers, and operating theaters, this mental discipline is essential.

The protective shield also helps doctors manage the cumulative impact of repeated exposure to suffering.

A physician may see dozens of patients in a single day, each carrying their own difficulties and fears. If the doctor attempted to emotionally absorb every situation, the psychological strain would grow rapidly. Detachment creates a boundary that prevents these experiences from overwhelming the physician's mental stability.

Many doctors describe this process as learning to compartmentalize.

Compartmentalization allows physicians to separate their professional experiences from their personal lives. A difficult case encountered during the day is placed mentally within a professional context rather than carried continuously into private moments. This separation helps doctors continue functioning without constant emotional exhaustion.

In this sense, detachment serves an important protective role.

It enables doctors to maintain consistency in their work. Patients benefit from physicians who remain calm, focused, and capable of making decisions under pressure. Emotional stability becomes part of professional reliability.

Yet the protective shield does not mean that doctors stop caring.

Behind the composed exterior, many physicians still feel the emotional impact of their work. They may remember certain patients long after treatment has ended. Some cases leave impressions that stay with them throughout their careers. The difference is that these feelings are often managed privately rather than expressed openly during clinical interactions.

The profession encourages this restraint because the doctor's primary responsibility is to provide effective care.

However, the shield of detachment also introduces a subtle risk. When the boundary becomes too strong, it can begin to isolate the doctor from the emotional dimension of the patient's experience. The protective mechanism that once allowed doctors to function effectively may gradually distance them from the people they treat.

This transition rarely occurs suddenly. It develops slowly as professional habits become deeply ingrained.

A doctor who consistently relies on detachment may begin to approach patient interactions primarily through clinical logic. Conversations may focus more on diagnosis and treatment than on emotional reassurance. The physician's attention remains directed toward solving medical problems.

From the doctor's perspective, this approach reflects professional discipline.

From the patient's perspective, however, the interaction may feel distant.

Understanding the protective shield of detachment therefore requires acknowledging both its necessity and its limitations. It allows doctors to endure the demands of their profession, but it must be balanced carefully to ensure that the human connection at the center of medicine does not fade behind the armor of professional control.

3.5 — When Protection Becomes Indifference

The emotional distance that doctors develop during their training begins as a protective skill. It helps them remain stable in environments filled with suffering, uncertainty, and urgent decisions. Without some level of emotional control, the psychological weight of the profession could easily overwhelm even the most dedicated physician.

But protective mechanisms in human behavior often carry a hidden risk: what begins as necessary adaptation can gradually become habit.

In medicine, this transition can occur so quietly that the doctor may not even notice it.

During the early years of practice, emotional distance is applied consciously. A doctor reminds themselves to remain calm while delivering difficult news. They focus deliberately on clinical reasoning rather than reacting emotionally to distressing situations. Detachment functions like a tool used when needed.

Over time, however, repeated use of this tool can reshape the doctor's natural response.

When a physician encounters hundreds or thousands of patients over the years, consultations start to follow recognizable patterns. Symptoms are described, examinations are performed, tests are reviewed, and treatment plans are recommended. Efficiency becomes essential because the number of patients waiting for care continues to grow.

The doctor learns to move through these interactions quickly and systematically.

From a clinical standpoint, this efficiency is valuable. It allows doctors to treat more patients, manage busy schedules, and maintain the pace required by modern healthcare systems. A physician who can evaluate symptoms quickly and make decisions with confidence becomes highly effective in such environments.

Yet the same efficiency can slowly narrow the emotional space within consultations.

Patients rarely experience their illness as routine. For them, the moment of visiting a doctor may carry anxiety, fear, or confusion. They may have spent days worrying about what their symptoms mean. Some may be facing medical uncertainty for the first time in their lives.

When these patients encounter a doctor who is moving rapidly through the consultation, the interaction may feel distant. The physician may appear focused entirely on medical data—symptoms, laboratory results, diagnostic possibilities—while the patient is still processing the emotional impact of being unwell.

This difference in perception creates a subtle gap.

For the doctor, the consultation is one among many in a demanding schedule. For the patient, it may be the most important conversation of the day.

If detachment becomes deeply ingrained, the doctor may begin to respond to patients primarily through clinical frameworks. Questions become shorter and more direct. Explanations may focus on technical details rather than reassurance. Conversations move quickly toward treatment decisions.

None of these actions necessarily reflect a lack of competence. The doctor may be diagnosing accurately and prescribing effective treatment.

But something in the interaction may feel incomplete.

Patients often notice when their concerns are addressed only at a technical level. Even brief signs of attentiveness—such as listening without interruption, acknowledging fear, or explaining a diagnosis carefully—can make a significant difference in how patients perceive their care.

When these elements disappear, patients may begin to feel that they are no longer seen as individuals but as cases passing through a system.

For doctors themselves, the transition from protective detachment to habitual distance may be difficult to recognize. The daily pressures of the profession leave little time for reflection. Consultations follow one another continuously, and the focus remains on solving medical problems rather than examining communication styles.

However, small signals sometimes reveal that the protective boundary has grown stronger than intended.

A doctor may notice impatience during consultations where patients speak at length. Emotional expressions from patients may feel uncomfortable or inconvenient. The physician may begin to rely almost entirely on clinical language when discussing illness.

These changes do not mean that the doctor has lost compassion. More often, they indicate the presence of emotional fatigue combined with professional routine.

The line between detachment and indifference is therefore not a sharp boundary but a gradual slope. Doctors move along it slowly, often without realizing how their professional habits are evolving.

Recognizing this possibility does not weaken the profession. On the contrary, it strengthens it.

Because awareness allows doctors to adjust their approach before the protective shield that once preserved their emotional stability becomes a barrier separating them from the people they are meant to serve.

3.6 — The Hidden Emotional Burden of Doctors

From the outside, doctors often appear composed, controlled, and professionally steady. Their conversations are structured, their decisions analytical, and their demeanor calm even in difficult situations. This image of emotional stability is one reason society places such trust in physicians. Patients expect doctors to remain confident when uncertainty arises and composed when circumstances become critical.

Yet behind this professional composure lies an emotional reality that is rarely discussed openly.

Doctors experience the same human responses to suffering that anyone else does. They feel concern when a patient deteriorates, frustration when treatments fail, and sadness when outcomes cannot be changed. The difference is that the profession requires these emotions to remain largely invisible during clinical practice.

Many physicians carry memories of specific patients long after treatment has ended.

Some remember the first patient they lost despite every effort made to save them. Others recall conversations with families who had to accept life-altering diagnoses. Certain cases leave a lasting impression not because they were medically complex, but because they revealed the fragile boundary between life and loss.

These experiences accumulate quietly over the years.

Unlike many professions where difficult events are occasional, medicine exposes doctors to emotionally challenging situations repeatedly. Delivering bad news, witnessing pain, managing emergencies, and facing unpredictable outcomes become regular parts of professional life.

Yet doctors are rarely given the opportunity to pause and process these experiences fully.

The structure of healthcare systems often leaves little space for reflection. After one difficult case ends, another patient requires attention. Clinical schedules continue. Documentation must be completed. The doctor moves forward because the system demands continuity.

As a result, emotional responses are often postponed rather than resolved.

Some physicians learn to carry these experiences privately. They may think about certain patients during quiet moments after work. Others discuss difficult cases with trusted colleagues who understand the unique pressures of medical practice. Within medical communities, these conversations sometimes serve as informal support systems.

However, the emotional burden of the profession often remains largely unspoken.

Medical culture has historically emphasized resilience and endurance. Doctors are expected to handle difficult situations without appearing overwhelmed. While this expectation reinforces professional stability, it can also discourage open acknowledgment of emotional strain.

Over time, this silence can create a hidden layer of psychological pressure.

Doctors may begin to feel responsible not only for their clinical decisions but also for outcomes that lie beyond their control. A patient's deterioration may raise quiet questions in the physician's mind: Was anything missed? Could something have been done differently?

Even when the medical care was appropriate, these thoughts can linger.

In addition to emotional challenges, physicians must also navigate the stress associated with responsibility. Medical decisions carry consequences that affect real lives. The awareness that a single judgment may influence a patient's future adds weight to everyday practice.

This constant responsibility, combined with repeated exposure to suffering, creates a form of emotional fatigue that is rarely visible to patients.

Some doctors respond by strengthening their emotional boundaries even further. Detachment becomes a way to prevent the accumulation of unresolved feelings. By focusing strictly on clinical tasks, the physician protects themselves from the emotional intensity of their work.

Yet the underlying burden does not always disappear.

It may surface unexpectedly—in moments of quiet reflection, during conversations with colleagues, or when a particular case resembles a past experience that left a strong impression. These moments remind doctors that beneath the professional exterior, they remain human beings processing the realities of illness, uncertainty, and loss.

Recognizing the hidden emotional burden carried by doctors is essential for understanding the full complexity of the profession.

The emotional distance that sometimes appears in clinical interactions is not always a sign of indifference. Often it reflects the invisible effort required to remain functional within a demanding environment where suffering is encountered daily.

Acknowledging this reality allows both doctors and patients to view the profession with greater understanding.

Because behind the white coat and the clinical language stands a person who, like everyone else, is learning how to navigate the emotional weight of human life and human fragility.

3.7 — Restoring Balance Without Losing Strength

If emotional detachment protects doctors from the overwhelming weight of their profession, the challenge that follows is how to maintain that protection without allowing it to become emotional disconnection. Medicine cannot function without composure and discipline, yet it also cannot fulfill its purpose if the human connection between doctor and patient disappears entirely.

The goal, therefore, is not to eliminate detachment but to balance it with awareness.

Doctors must remain capable of performing under pressure. A physician facing a critical patient cannot afford to become emotionally immobilized. Clinical reasoning, steady hands, and clear thinking must guide treatment decisions. The scientific side of medicine requires mental focus that is not disrupted by intense emotional reaction.

However, maintaining professional strength does not mean abandoning empathy.

Over time, experienced doctors often discover that compassion does not always require emotional immersion. It can exist in quieter forms—listening carefully, acknowledging uncertainty honestly, or offering reassurance during difficult moments. These gestures do not slow the clinical process, but they remind patients that the doctor recognizes their vulnerability.

Professional maturity in medicine often lies in learning this balance.

Young doctors sometimes believe they must choose between two extremes: emotional involvement that becomes overwhelming or detachment that becomes distant. With experience, many physicians realize that there is a middle ground where empathy and objectivity coexist.

In this balanced approach, the doctor continues to analyze symptoms and follow clinical protocols, but remains aware that every diagnosis affects a person's life beyond the hospital setting. The physician speaks with clarity but also with respect for the emotional reality the patient may be experiencing.

Communication plays a crucial role in maintaining this balance.

Patients rarely expect doctors to share their emotional burden completely. What they often seek is recognition that their concerns are being heard and understood. A brief explanation of a diagnosis, a moment taken to answer a question, or a calm acknowledgment of the patient's fear can transform the tone of the interaction.

Such communication does not require additional medical knowledge. It requires awareness.

Doctors who maintain this awareness often find that it strengthens rather than weakens their professional role. Patients who feel understood are more likely to trust medical advice, follow treatment plans, and cooperate during recovery. The relationship between doctor and patient becomes collaborative rather than purely procedural.

Restoring balance also involves recognizing the importance of self-awareness among physicians.

Doctors who occasionally reflect on their own emotional responses are better able to identify when detachment has become excessive. A physician who notices impatience during consultations or emotional numbness toward patient suffering may recognize that fatigue or burnout is influencing their behavior.

In such moments, reflection becomes a form of professional maintenance.

Just as medical knowledge must be updated regularly, emotional awareness must also be renewed over time. Some doctors achieve this through conversations with colleagues, mentorship, or simply through quiet reflection on their experiences.

The profession itself benefits when such awareness is encouraged rather than suppressed.

Ultimately, restoring balance does not require dramatic changes in how medicine is practiced. It requires remembering that clinical skill and human understanding are not opposing forces. They are complementary aspects of the same profession.

A doctor can remain scientifically rigorous while still recognizing the human context of illness.

The protective strength developed through training does not need to disappear. It simply needs to remain flexible enough to allow moments of connection to emerge when patients need them most.

In this way, the emotional discipline of medicine becomes not a barrier between doctor and patient, but a framework within which compassion can continue to exist without overwhelming the physician who must carry the responsibility of healing.

The Human Behind the White Coat

The image of a doctor that society often carries is one of certainty and control. The white coat, the calm voice, the confident diagnosis—these symbols suggest a person who stands firmly above the uncertainty of illness. Patients approach doctors expecting clarity, stability, and answers during moments when their own lives feel fragile.

Yet behind this professional image stands a human being navigating the emotional realities of a demanding profession.

Doctors spend years learning how to think clearly in the presence of suffering. They develop the ability to manage difficult situations without allowing emotion to disrupt judgment. This discipline is not accidental; it is necessary. Without it, the profession would become impossible to sustain.

But emotional control should not be mistaken for emotional absence.

The physician who appears composed during a consultation may carry memories of patients whose stories left a lasting impression. Certain cases remain vivid even years later—moments when recovery occurred against the odds, or when medicine reached its limits despite every effort made.

These experiences form part of the doctor's inner landscape, even when they are rarely spoken aloud.

At the same time, patients often encounter doctors only during brief moments of interaction. They see the clinical focus, the structured questions, and the efficient movement of the consultation. What remains hidden is the emotional discipline that allows the physician to maintain this stability.

This difference in perspective can easily lead to misunderstanding.

Patients may interpret emotional restraint as indifference, while doctors may believe they are simply fulfilling their professional responsibilities. In reality, both sides are responding to the same situation from different positions.

The patient stands within the uncertainty of illness.

The doctor stands within the responsibility of managing it.

Recognizing this distinction is essential for rebuilding trust within modern healthcare. Doctors are not immune to the emotional weight of their work, and patients are not merely medical conditions awaiting treatment. Both exist within a shared moment where vulnerability meets responsibility.

The white coat represents knowledge and authority, but it also conceals the effort required to carry these responsibilities day after day.

Behind it stands a person who must continually balance clinical discipline with human awareness. A person who must remain steady when others feel fear. A person who must accept that medicine, despite all its progress, cannot always provide the outcomes everyone hopes for.

Understanding the emotional cost of this balance allows the profession to be seen more honestly.

Doctors are neither detached machines nor flawless healers. They are individuals who have learned to navigate one of the most emotionally demanding roles in society.

And perhaps the most important step toward restoring the human connection in medicine begins with acknowledging this simple truth: before the white coat became a symbol of authority, it was worn by someone who was learning how to carry the weight of another person's life with both knowledge and restraint.

Chapter 4 — The Silent Burnout

The Fatigue No One Talks About

There is a kind of exhaustion in medicine that rarely appears in medical reports, hospital statistics, or public conversations. It does not come from a single long shift or a particularly difficult day in the ward. Instead, it grows slowly over time—through years of responsibility, constant decision-making, and the quiet awareness that every choice made in the profession carries real consequences.

From the outside, doctors often appear composed and capable. They move confidently through hospital corridors, review reports, speak with patients, and make treatment decisions with steady professionalism. To patients and families, the doctor represents clarity in moments of uncertainty. The white coat symbolizes knowledge, authority, and reliability.

What remains less visible is the mental landscape behind that composed exterior.

Every consultation requires attention. Every diagnosis requires judgment. Even routine cases involve evaluating symptoms, considering possible conditions, reviewing previous medical history, and deciding whether further investigation is necessary. These decisions may seem ordinary to observers, but for the doctor they accumulate into a continuous stream of responsibility.

Over the course of a day, a physician may make dozens of clinical judgments. Some are straightforward, but others carry uncertainty. Should a test be ordered now or later? Is a symptom minor or a sign of something serious? Is the treatment sufficient, or should it be adjusted?

Each decision requires concentration, and each one carries potential consequences.

Unlike many professions where decisions can be revisited without major impact, medical decisions affect real lives. A correct judgment can lead to recovery. A delayed or incorrect one may complicate treatment. Even when doctors act carefully and responsibly, the awareness of this possibility remains in the background of their thinking.

This constant mental engagement creates a unique form of fatigue.

It is not always physical tiredness, though long working hours contribute to it. It is the cumulative strain of sustained responsibility—the knowledge that the profession does not allow casual decisions or emotional distraction.

At the same time, the healthcare environment rarely pauses.

Hospitals operate continuously. Patients arrive at all hours. Emergencies interrupt routines without warning. A difficult case may be followed immediately by another patient requiring attention. The doctor moves from one situation to the next because the system demands continuity.

Within this rhythm, there is often little time to step back and recognize the gradual accumulation of pressure.

Many doctors continue working with efficiency even as the mental load increases. They remain professional, attentive, and capable. Yet beneath this steady performance lies a fatigue that is rarely acknowledged openly.

It is not dramatic or sudden. It does not announce itself loudly. Instead, it grows quietly through years of carrying responsibility that few outside the profession fully understand.

This is the silent burnout of medicine—the exhaustion that develops not from a lack of dedication, but from the weight of sustaining it every day.

4.1 — The Weight of Continuous Decisions

Every profession requires decisions, but few professions require them with the frequency and consequence that medicine does. From the moment a doctor begins the day's work, the mind enters a continuous cycle of evaluation, judgment, and action.

A patient walks into the clinic and describes symptoms. Within seconds, the doctor's mind begins sorting possibilities. Is the complaint minor, or could it indicate something more serious? Are the symptoms consistent with a known condition, or do they require further investigation? Should treatment begin immediately, or should additional tests be ordered first?

Each of these questions leads to a decision.

Some decisions appear small on the surface—prescribing medication, ordering a diagnostic test, recommending rest or follow-up observation. Yet each one carries implications. A medication may relieve symptoms but also carry side effects. A test may confirm a diagnosis but also impose financial cost or emotional anxiety for the patient.

The doctor must weigh these possibilities quickly and carefully.

Over the course of a single consultation, dozens of micro-decisions take place: interpreting symptoms, choosing examination methods, evaluating previous medical history, considering risk factors, and determining the most appropriate course of action. When multiplied across many patients in a single day, this process becomes mentally demanding.

A physician in a busy clinic may see twenty, thirty, or even more patients within a few hours. Each patient arrives with a unique situation requiring fresh attention. The doctor cannot rely entirely on routine responses. Every case demands evaluation, even when symptoms appear familiar.

This constant switching of attention creates what psychologists describe as decision fatigue.

Decision fatigue occurs when the mind becomes tired from making repeated judgments without sufficient time to recover. In medicine, the consequences of such fatigue can be significant. Doctors must remain alert even when mentally tired because the next decision may involve a critical diagnosis.

For this reason, physicians learn to develop structured methods of thinking.

Clinical frameworks, diagnostic guidelines, and treatment protocols help reduce the mental burden of repeated decision-making. By organizing information systematically, doctors can process cases more efficiently and reduce the risk of oversight.

Yet even with these tools, the cognitive load remains substantial.

Consider the physician working in an emergency department. Within a single shift, they may encounter patients with chest pain, injuries from accidents, infections, allergic reactions, and numerous other conditions. Each case demands immediate attention and a clear judgment about urgency.

The doctor must constantly prioritize: which patient requires treatment first, which symptoms signal danger, which conditions can safely wait for further evaluation.

This environment requires rapid mental adjustment. The physician's attention moves from one medical scenario to another without pause.

Outside observers may see only the visible actions—the examination, the prescription, the brief explanation given to the patient. What remains unseen is the mental process unfolding continuously in the background.

The doctor is evaluating probabilities, anticipating complications, recalling medical knowledge, and comparing current symptoms with past experiences. Even routine consultations involve layers of analysis that remain invisible to patients.

Over time, the accumulation of these decisions begins to weigh on the mind.

Unlike tasks that involve physical repetition, clinical decisions cannot become entirely automatic. Every patient introduces new variables. The doctor must remain mentally present, regardless of fatigue or external distractions.

This constant demand for judgment becomes one of the defining pressures of the profession.

It is also one of the least visible.

Patients rarely see the hundreds of decisions a doctor makes throughout the day. They see only the final recommendation given during their consultation. Yet behind that single recommendation lies a chain of reasoning shaped by experience, knowledge, and careful consideration.

The weight of continuous decisions therefore becomes an invisible companion in the life of a doctor—present from the first patient of the morning to the last case of the day.

And unlike many other forms of work, the mind does not always switch off when the hospital doors close. The responsibility attached to those decisions often travels home with the physician, quietly extending the mental demands of the profession beyond the clinic itself.

4.2 — Responsibility That Never Fully Ends

One of the defining characteristics of medical practice is responsibility—responsibility that does not always end when the working day finishes. In many professions, a task completed during office hours can be set aside once the day is over. A report submitted, a meeting concluded, or a project delivered allows the mind to close that chapter and move on.

Medicine rarely provides that kind of closure.

A doctor's decisions are connected to outcomes that continue unfolding long after the consultation ends. A treatment prescribed in the morning may determine whether a patient recovers over the next few days. A diagnosis made during a brief examination may influence a patient's life for months or even years.

This awareness stays with the physician.

When doctors leave the hospital or clinic, their work does not completely disappear from their thoughts. Many physicians find themselves reflecting on cases they handled during the day. Did the diagnosis fully explain the symptoms? Was the chosen treatment the most appropriate option? Should additional tests have been ordered?

These questions often arise not because the doctor made a mistake, but because the profession encourages constant vigilance.

Medical training emphasizes the importance of careful judgment. Students are taught that overlooking a detail can have serious consequences. As a result, doctors develop the habit of reviewing their decisions mentally, even when they have acted responsibly and according to established medical knowledge.

This ongoing reflection becomes part of professional life.

Some cases remain in the mind because they are complex or unusual. Others linger because the patient's condition was uncertain at the time of consultation. A doctor may wonder how a particular patient is responding to treatment or whether the symptoms might evolve in unexpected ways.

Even experienced physicians sometimes carry such thoughts beyond the hospital environment.

The sense of responsibility becomes particularly intense in situations where outcomes are unpredictable. A patient admitted in critical condition, a diagnosis that must be confirmed through further testing, or a treatment that requires close monitoring can create a lingering awareness that the situation is not fully resolved.

For doctors working in hospitals, this responsibility often continues through on-call duties.

Even after leaving the ward, physicians may remain reachable by phone in case a patient's condition changes. A late-night call about a complication or emergency reminds the doctor that the boundaries between personal time and professional responsibility are not always clearly defined.

This constant connection to patient care can make it difficult for doctors to detach completely from their work.

Beyond clinical responsibility, there is also the ethical dimension of medical practice. Doctors are aware that patients trust them with deeply personal concerns and rely on their expertise during moments of vulnerability. This trust carries moral weight.

When a patient shares fears about illness or places hope in a treatment plan, the doctor becomes part of a situation that extends beyond technical medicine. The physician must not only apply knowledge correctly but also ensure that decisions are made with care and honesty.

Carrying this responsibility day after day can become mentally demanding.

Many doctors continue reflecting on their cases because they genuinely want the best possible outcomes for their patients. This commitment often motivates them to study further, consult colleagues, or review medical literature when faced with challenging situations.

But it also means that the profession does not easily allow emotional distance from responsibility.

A doctor may leave the hospital physically, but the awareness of patients and their conditions often remains present in the background of the mind. Conversations with family or quiet moments at home may occasionally be interrupted by thoughts about cases handled earlier in the day.

Over time, this constant sense of responsibility becomes part of the doctor's identity.

It reflects dedication to the profession, but it also contributes to the silent fatigue that many physicians experience. The mind remains engaged with medical decisions even when the workday has officially ended.

For the public, the image of a doctor often centers on the consultation room or the hospital ward. Yet the responsibility carried by doctors extends far beyond these visible settings.

It follows them quietly, shaping how they think, reflect, and rest—even when no patient is physically present.

4.3 — The System That Never Sleeps

Unlike many professions that operate within fixed schedules, healthcare functions without interruption. Hospitals remain active twenty-four hours a day, every day of the year. Illness does not pause for weekends, holidays, or personal convenience. Accidents happen at midnight, complications arise at dawn, and emergencies arrive without warning.

For doctors working within this environment, the rhythm of life becomes closely tied to the rhythm of the healthcare system.

During medical training, this reality begins to take shape through long shifts and irregular schedules. Interns and residents often experience extended working hours that move beyond the structure of ordinary workdays. Night duties become routine. A shift that begins in the evening may continue until the following morning, sometimes longer when emergencies occur.

Sleep becomes fragmented and unpredictable.

A resident may leave the hospital after a night shift only to return again the next day for clinical rounds or academic responsibilities.

The body's natural cycle of rest and recovery often struggles to adjust to these patterns. Over time, sleep deprivation becomes an almost normalized part of the profession.

This lack of consistent rest has consequences that extend beyond physical tiredness.

The human brain depends on adequate sleep to maintain cognitive clarity and emotional stability. When sleep becomes irregular, concentration becomes more difficult, and the mind must work harder to maintain the same level of performance. Doctors must remain attentive even when their bodies are signaling fatigue.

In high-pressure environments such as emergency departments or intensive care units, this challenge becomes particularly visible.

A physician may need to assess a critically ill patient in the middle of the night after several hours of continuous work. Despite exhaustion, the doctor must evaluate symptoms, interpret data, and initiate treatment with the same accuracy expected during the day.

This expectation forms part of the professional culture of medicine.

Doctors are trained to endure demanding schedules because patient care requires constant availability. The healthcare system relies on physicians who can respond to emergencies regardless of the hour. In this sense, endurance becomes a professional virtue.

However, the culture of endurance also carries hidden costs.

Long hours and irregular schedules gradually affect the doctor's mental and physical well-being. Fatigue accumulates quietly, sometimes becoming noticeable only after months or years of demanding work patterns. Even when doctors adapt to these conditions, the body and mind continue to experience strain.

In addition to clinical duties, many physicians must also manage administrative responsibilities, academic obligations, and ongoing professional development. Medical knowledge evolves rapidly, requiring doctors to stay updated with new research, guidelines, and technologies.

This constant demand for learning adds another layer of pressure to an already demanding schedule.

Outside the hospital, personal life often adjusts around professional responsibilities. Family events, social gatherings, and periods of rest may be interrupted by unexpected calls or urgent situations requiring the doctor's attention. The boundaries between professional and personal time become fluid.

Over time, many physicians come to accept this reality as part of the profession they chose.

Yet the continuous nature of the healthcare system means that doctors rarely experience complete mental disengagement from their work. Even when they are physically away from the hospital, the possibility of being called back or consulted about a patient remains present.

This persistent connection to responsibility contributes to the silent fatigue described earlier in the chapter.

The system that never sleeps requires doctors who remain mentally alert despite long hours, irregular rest, and constant responsibility. While many physicians manage these demands with dedication and resilience, the cumulative strain can gradually shape how they experience their work.

Understanding this aspect of medical life reveals an important truth: the pressures faced by doctors are not only created by individual cases or difficult decisions. They are also built into the structure of a profession that operates continuously in service of human health.

4.4 — The Fear of Error

Few responsibilities weigh as heavily as the possibility of making a mistake when another person's life may be affected by the outcome.

In medicine, this awareness accompanies doctors from the earliest stages of training and remains present throughout their careers.

Every physician understands that clinical decisions must be made with care and precision. A diagnosis must be accurate. A medication must be prescribed in the correct dosage. A procedure must be performed with attention to detail. Even routine tasks require concentration because small oversights can sometimes lead to larger consequences.

This constant need for accuracy creates a unique psychological pressure.

Unlike many fields where errors can be corrected with minimal impact, mistakes in medicine can have immediate and serious effects. A missed symptom might delay treatment. A misinterpretation of test results might lead to an incorrect diagnosis. Even when such situations are rare, the possibility remains in the doctor's mind.

Doctors therefore develop a deep awareness of risk.

Clinical training emphasizes careful observation and verification. Students are taught to double-check findings, review patient histories thoroughly, and consult colleagues when uncertainty arises. This culture of caution helps reduce errors, but it also reinforces the understanding that medicine demands continuous vigilance.

During busy clinical days, the physician's mind remains alert to potential problems.

While examining a patient, the doctor may consider several possible diagnoses simultaneously, evaluating which one fits the symptoms most closely. While reviewing laboratory results, the physician may search for patterns that confirm or challenge initial impressions. Even when the case appears straightforward, doctors often remain cautious because unusual presentations can occur.

This mental habit of constantly questioning one's conclusions is part of responsible medical practice.

However, the need for such vigilance also contributes to psychological strain. Doctors know that the consequences of error extend beyond professional embarrassment. A medical mistake may affect a patient's health, alter a treatment plan, or in severe cases lead to irreversible outcomes.

For physicians who take their responsibilities seriously, this possibility is never taken lightly.

Many doctors therefore develop the practice of reviewing their decisions mentally, sometimes even after the consultation has ended. They may revisit a diagnosis to ensure that no important symptom was overlooked. They may reconsider whether additional tests should have been ordered.

Such reflection often arises from professional commitment rather than insecurity.

At the same time, the environment of modern healthcare has intensified awareness of medical error. Advances in technology allow detailed monitoring of clinical decisions. Hospital systems maintain extensive documentation. Professional guidelines define recommended procedures for many conditions.

These developments improve patient safety but also increase scrutiny of the physician's work.

Doctors know that their decisions may later be reviewed by colleagues, institutions, or regulatory bodies. This awareness encourages careful practice but can also create additional stress, particularly in situations where medical uncertainty is unavoidable.

Because despite all scientific progress, medicine remains a field where complete certainty is rarely possible.

Symptoms can overlap between conditions. Test results may not always provide clear answers. Some illnesses develop gradually, revealing their full nature only over time. In such situations, doctors must make the best possible decision with the information available at that moment.

Living with this uncertainty is one of the less visible challenges of the profession.

The fear of error does not mean that doctors constantly doubt their abilities. Most physicians develop confidence through training and experience. Yet even the most experienced doctors remain aware that medicine requires humility.

Each patient presents a new situation. Each case carries the possibility of unexpected developments.

This awareness keeps doctors attentive and careful. But it also adds another layer to the silent burnout described in this chapter—the mental pressure of knowing that every decision must be made with the utmost responsibility, even in the face of uncertainty.

4.5 — Medicine Under Legal Scrutiny

Medicine today does not operate only within the domain of science and clinical judgment. It also functions within a legal and regulatory framework that influences how doctors practice their profession. While these structures exist to protect patients and ensure accountability, they also introduce a new dimension of pressure that many doctors must navigate carefully.

In earlier decades, the relationship between doctor and patient relied heavily on trust. Medical decisions were largely accepted based on the physician's expertise, and legal disputes were relatively uncommon. Over time, however, healthcare systems around the world have become more complex, and patient awareness of legal rights has increased significantly.

This shift has brought important benefits. Greater accountability helps maintain standards of care and protects patients from negligence. Transparent systems encourage careful documentation and responsible clinical practice. Yet the same environment has also made many doctors more conscious of the possibility that their decisions may later be examined in legal contexts.

Every diagnosis, prescription, and procedure must now be recorded with precision.

Doctors spend considerable time documenting consultations, test results, and treatment decisions in medical records. These records serve not only as clinical references but also as legal documents that demonstrate how decisions were made. A well-documented case can protect both patient and physician by providing a clear record of the reasoning behind medical actions.

However, the necessity of such documentation adds to the already demanding workload of physicians.

In busy clinical environments, doctors may find themselves balancing patient interaction with the need to complete extensive paperwork or electronic records. While documentation improves accountability, it can also reduce the time available for direct communication with patients.

Beyond documentation, there is also the psychological awareness that medical decisions may be questioned in the future.

A patient's condition might evolve unexpectedly. A treatment may not produce the desired outcome. Even when a doctor has acted responsibly and according to accepted medical guidelines, the possibility of legal scrutiny remains present.

This awareness can subtly influence how doctors approach their work.

Some physicians begin practicing what is often called defensive medicine. Instead of relying solely on clinical judgment, they may order additional tests or procedures primarily to ensure that no possibility is overlooked. While such caution may provide reassurance, it can also increase costs and extend the complexity of care.

Defensive medicine reflects a broader shift in the medical environment: doctors must consider not only what is medically appropriate but also how their decisions might be interpreted later by regulatory bodies, hospital administrations, or legal authorities.

This situation places physicians in a delicate position.

On one hand, they must act quickly and confidently to treat patients effectively. On the other, they must remain aware that every action could later be analyzed with the benefit of hindsight. Decisions made in moments of uncertainty may be evaluated later as if all information had been available at the time.

For many doctors, this possibility creates an additional layer of mental strain.

It reinforces the feeling that the profession operates under constant observation. Even experienced physicians who practice carefully may feel the pressure of ensuring that every step of their decision-making process is thoroughly documented and defensible.

Despite these challenges, most doctors accept the need for legal accountability as part of modern healthcare. Responsible medical practice requires transparency and adherence to established standards. Patients deserve protection from negligence, and healthcare systems must maintain trust.

However, understanding the legal dimension of medicine also reveals why the psychological burden on doctors continues to grow.

Clinical decisions are no longer judged solely by their medical intent or reasoning. They must also withstand scrutiny from administrative and legal perspectives. The physician must think simultaneously as a clinician, a communicator, and at times a cautious record keeper.

This constant awareness of legal responsibility becomes another silent contributor to the fatigue many doctors experience.

It reminds them that every consultation involves not only the challenge of diagnosing illness but also the need to navigate a complex environment where science, ethics, and law intersect.

4.6 — Emotional Exhaustion Without Recognition

Burnout in medicine rarely appears suddenly or dramatically. It does not always begin with a clear moment when a doctor realizes that something has changed. Instead, it develops quietly over time, often unnoticed even by the physicians experiencing it.

In many cases, a doctor continues to perform effectively while burnout slowly takes root beneath the surface.

From the outside, the physician appears the same—consultations continue, clinical decisions are made, and patients receive treatment. The doctor may still speak confidently, complete duties responsibly, and maintain professional composure. Yet internally, the experience of practicing medicine may begin to feel different.

Tasks that once carried a sense of purpose may start to feel mechanical. Conversations with patients may feel routine rather than meaningful. The energy required to maintain the same level of attentiveness gradually increases.

This is the beginning of emotional exhaustion.

Emotional exhaustion occurs when the mind becomes fatigued from sustained responsibility, constant vigilance, and repeated exposure to stressful situations. In medicine, these conditions are present almost every day. Doctors must remain attentive to symptoms, cautious about errors, responsive to emergencies, and sensitive to the needs of patients and families.

Over time, this constant engagement drains mental energy.

One of the subtle signs of burnout is emotional numbness. A doctor who once reacted strongly to difficult situations may begin to feel less affected by them. At first, this numbness may seem helpful because it reduces the emotional intensity of the work. However, it can also signal that the physician's psychological resources are becoming depleted.

Another common sign is reduced motivation.

Doctors who entered the profession with enthusiasm and dedication may begin to feel that their work has become repetitive or overwhelming. The sense of accomplishment that once accompanied successful treatment may become less noticeable as fatigue grows.

Yet many physicians do not openly discuss these experiences.

Medical culture has traditionally valued resilience and endurance. Doctors are trained to remain composed and to continue working even when conditions are demanding. As a result, admitting emotional fatigue may feel uncomfortable or even inappropriate within professional environments.

Some physicians worry that acknowledging burnout might be interpreted as weakness or lack of commitment. Others simply feel that there is little time to address their own well-being while patients continue to require care.

Consequently, burnout often remains invisible.

Colleagues may notice only subtle changes—a quieter demeanor, shorter interactions with patients, or a sense that the doctor appears constantly tired. Even these signals may be overlooked in busy hospital settings where many professionals are experiencing similar pressures.

The invisibility of burnout makes it particularly difficult to address.

Because the doctor continues to function, the underlying exhaustion may not receive attention until it becomes severe. In some cases, physicians begin to distance themselves emotionally from their work as a coping mechanism. Detachment becomes stronger, conversations become shorter, and the human connection with patients gradually weakens.

Ironically, this distancing may further deepen the sense of isolation.

Doctors who entered the profession with a strong desire to help people may begin to feel disconnected from the very purpose that once motivated them. The profession that once inspired pride may begin to feel like a series of responsibilities that must simply be managed.

Understanding emotional exhaustion is essential to understanding the silent burnout described in this chapter.

Burnout does not mean that doctors have lost their competence or their commitment. More often, it reflects the cumulative effect of carrying responsibilities that are emotionally demanding, cognitively intense, and sustained over long periods without sufficient recognition or support.

Behind the composed exterior of many physicians lies a quiet fatigue—one that develops not from a lack of dedication, but from the effort required to maintain it day after day.

4.7 — Recovering Stability in a Demanding Profession

Recognizing burnout is only the first step. The more important challenge is understanding how doctors can restore balance without losing the professional strength that medicine requires. The goal is not to reduce commitment or responsibility, but to ensure that the physician's capacity to carry those responsibilities remains sustainable over time.

Medicine is a demanding profession, and it will likely remain so. Patients will continue to depend on doctors during moments of vulnerability, and the healthcare system will continue to require long hours, careful judgment, and constant vigilance. Yet acknowledging the pressures faced by doctors opens the possibility of creating healthier ways to navigate them.

One important step is awareness.

Many physicians become so accustomed to the pace and intensity of their work that they stop noticing the gradual accumulation of fatigue. Recognizing early signs of burnout—persistent exhaustion, emotional numbness, irritability, or reduced motivation—can help doctors address the problem before it becomes overwhelming.

Self-awareness allows physicians to pause and evaluate how their professional responsibilities are affecting their mental and emotional well-being.

Another essential factor is the role of institutional support.

Hospitals and healthcare systems rely heavily on the dedication of doctors, yet the well-being of these professionals has not always received sufficient attention. Work schedules, staffing levels, and administrative demands all influence the stress experienced by physicians. When healthcare institutions recognize that doctor well-being directly affects patient care, they can begin to design systems that support both.

Adequate rest periods, reasonable workloads, and environments that encourage open discussion of professional challenges can significantly reduce the risk of burnout.

Equally important is the culture within the medical community itself.

Doctors often feel more comfortable discussing difficulties with colleagues who understand the unique pressures of the profession. Informal conversations between physicians can provide valuable emotional support. Sharing experiences—whether about challenging cases, ethical dilemmas, or personal fatigue—helps normalize the reality that even the most capable doctors face moments of strain.

These conversations remind physicians that they are not alone in their experiences.

Professional reflection also plays a role in restoring stability.

Some doctors find that taking time to reflect on why they entered medicine helps reconnect them with the deeper meaning of their work. The profession is not defined only by long hours and difficult decisions; it also includes moments of recovery, gratitude from patients, and the satisfaction of helping someone regain health.

Remembering these moments can restore a sense of purpose that counters the fatigue of routine responsibilities.

Maintaining balance also requires attention to life outside the hospital.

Doctors who preserve time for family, personal interests, and rest often find that these experiences help restore emotional energy. Engaging in activities unrelated to medicine allows the mind to step away from clinical responsibilities, creating space for recovery.

While such balance is not always easy to achieve, it remains essential for long-term sustainability in the profession.

Ultimately, recovering stability does not mean reducing the seriousness with which doctors approach their work. Instead, it means recognizing that caring for others requires maintaining the capacity to care.

A physician who remains mentally and emotionally healthy is better equipped to provide thoughtful and attentive care to patients. Strength in medicine is not defined only by endurance but also by the ability to sustain compassion and clarity over time.

In this way, addressing burnout becomes not only a matter of personal well-being but also a matter of professional responsibility.

Because the health of the healthcare system depends not only on the treatments it provides but also on the well-being of the people entrusted with delivering those treatments.

The Strength That Needs Care

Society often views doctors through a particular lens. They are expected to be resilient, composed, and endlessly capable of carrying responsibility. The white coat symbolizes knowledge and authority, but it also creates an impression that doctors themselves are immune to the pressures they face.

In reality, the profession asks physicians to sustain a level of responsibility that few other roles require.

Every day, doctors stand at the intersection of uncertainty and expectation. Patients arrive seeking answers, relief, and reassurance. Families look to the physician for guidance during moments of fear. Hospitals rely on doctors to maintain the functioning of complex healthcare systems.

Amid all of this, the doctor must remain steady.

This steadiness often leads others to assume that doctors are unaffected by the emotional and mental demands of their work. The quiet fatigue, the weight of decisions, and the accumulation of difficult experiences remain largely invisible behind professional composure.

Yet strength in medicine does not mean the absence of vulnerability.

Doctors are human beings who must continuously process the realities of illness, suffering, and responsibility. They witness moments that most people encounter only rarely—life-changing diagnoses, unexpected recoveries, and sometimes the limits of medical intervention.

Carrying these experiences day after day requires extraordinary endurance.

But endurance alone is not enough.

A healthcare system that depends on doctors must also recognize the importance of supporting them. When physicians become overwhelmed or emotionally exhausted, the quality of care inevitably suffers. Patients benefit most when doctors remain not only knowledgeable and skilled but also mentally and emotionally balanced.

Caring for doctors therefore becomes part of caring for patients.

This understanding requires a shift in perspective—from seeing burnout as an individual weakness to recognizing it as a signal that the demands placed on the profession have reached unsustainable levels. Addressing these pressures requires attention from institutions, colleagues, and the broader healthcare culture.

Doctors themselves also play a role in maintaining this balance. Acknowledging fatigue, reflecting on experiences, and seeking support when needed are not signs of weakness. They are acts of professional responsibility.

Because medicine is not sustained by knowledge alone. It is sustained by people who are willing to carry the responsibility of healing others.

The strength of the profession lies not in denying the pressures doctors face, but in recognizing that even those who care for others must also be cared for.

Only when this truth is accepted can the profession remain both humane and sustainable—for doctors and for the patients who depend on them.

Reflective Interlude

Between Illness and Humanity

Up to this point, we have looked closely at the inner landscape of the doctor. The long training, the emotional distance, the silent burnout, the weight of decisions, and the invisible pressure carried by those who practice medicine. These chapters reveal a reality that patients rarely see—the human cost of standing on the side of responsibility.

But medicine does not exist only within the mind of the doctor.

It unfolds within a larger field of human experience.

Every consultation is not merely a clinical event where symptoms are examined and treatments prescribed. It is a meeting point between two human realities. One person arrives carrying illness, uncertainty, and vulnerability. The other arrives carrying knowledge, responsibility, and professional discipline.

Between these two individuals lies something deeper than a medical transaction.

A patient does not walk into a clinic as a biological organism alone. Behind the symptoms lies a story. There may be fear about the future, anxiety about medical expenses, pressure from family members, or the quiet burden of social expectations. Sometimes the illness is not only physical; it is woven into the person's life circumstances.

The doctor, standing on the other side of the consultation table, must navigate all of this within a limited window of time.

In medical textbooks, diseases appear in clear descriptions—symptoms, causes, treatments. In real life, however, illness rarely arrives in such orderly form. It enters the consultation room surrounded by emotions, relationships, and practical concerns that extend far beyond the boundaries of biology.

This is where medicine reveals its deeper complexity.

A doctor may prescribe the correct treatment, yet recovery also depends on factors that lie outside the prescription. Can the patient afford the medication? Does the family support the treatment plan? Is the patient emotionally prepared to follow medical advice?

Health care therefore becomes more than the management of disease.

It becomes a dynamic interaction between individuals, institutions, and society. Doctors, patients, families, hospitals, and communities all participate in shaping the outcome of medical care. Each plays a role, consciously or unconsciously, in determining whether treatment succeeds or fails.

Within this dynamic field, doctors occupy a particularly important position.

Patients often approach physicians during moments of uncertainty when trust becomes essential. The doctor's words can calm anxiety or amplify it. A simple explanation can restore confidence, while a rushed interaction can create confusion. The doctor's presence therefore influences not only medical decisions but also the emotional environment surrounding illness.

Yet this delicate balance of trust is becoming increasingly fragile.

Across many healthcare systems, tensions between doctors and patients are growing. Patients sometimes feel unheard or misunderstood. Doctors sometimes feel accused or unfairly judged. Miscommunication, systemic pressures, and rising expectations from both sides are slowly eroding the trust that once formed the foundation of medical relationships.

Understanding this shift requires looking beyond individual behavior.

The problem is rarely caused by doctors alone or by patients alone. It emerges from the interaction of multiple forces—social expectations, economic pressures, institutional constraints, and the emotional vulnerability that illness brings.

In the next part of this book, we move from the inner world of doctors to the shared human field in which medicine actually operates.

Because healing is never produced by knowledge alone.

It emerges from a complex web of participation where science, trust, responsibility, and human experience meet in the same moment—the moment when a doctor and a patient sit across from each other, trying to find a path back to health.

PART II — THE HUMAN FIELD OF MEDICINE

Disease may be biological, but healing always exists within a human context.

Chapter 5 — The Patient Beyond Biology

The Person Behind the Symptoms

In clinical practice, medicine often begins with a set of observable facts. A patient arrives with symptoms, the doctor asks structured questions, conducts an examination, and attempts to identify the biological cause of the problem. The process is logical and necessary. Diagnosis depends on recognizing patterns in the body—changes in organs, tissues, or chemical processes that signal disease.

Yet the person who enters the consultation room is never just a biological system.

Behind the symptoms stands an individual whose life has already been affected by the possibility of illness. Before meeting the doctor, the patient may have spent hours or days worrying about what the symptoms mean. A persistent pain, unusual fatigue, or unexplained change in health often triggers a chain of thoughts that extend far beyond the physical discomfort itself.

Questions begin to form quietly in the mind.

Is this serious? Will it affect my ability to work? What will happen to my family if the diagnosis is severe?

These concerns rarely appear in medical records, but they are present in the patient's experience long before the doctor begins the examination.

Illness does not enter a person's life in isolation. It touches relationships, responsibilities, and personal identity. A parent may worry about who will care for their children if treatment requires hospitalization. A worker may fear losing income during recovery. Someone supporting an extended family may feel pressure to continue functioning despite worsening symptoms.

The disease therefore becomes intertwined with the patient's social reality.

Even when the illness itself is medically manageable, the surrounding circumstances may amplify the patient's distress. Financial concerns, family expectations, cultural beliefs, and personal fears all shape how a patient experiences the condition.

For the doctor, however, the consultation begins at a different point.

The physician encounters the patient at the moment when symptoms are presented and clinical evaluation begins. The doctor must focus on identifying the biological problem and determining the appropriate treatment. This focus is essential because accurate diagnosis is the foundation of effective medicine.

But if the consultation remains limited only to biological analysis, an important dimension of the patient's experience may remain unseen.

Two patients with the same diagnosis may experience their illness in completely different ways. One may approach treatment calmly, supported by family and financial stability. Another may face the same condition with fear, isolation, or uncertainty about how treatment will affect their livelihood.

The disease may be identical, but the human context is entirely different.

Understanding this difference does not mean that doctors must solve every social or emotional challenge faced by their patients. Medicine cannot eliminate all the difficulties that illness brings into a person's life.

What it can do, however, is acknowledge that these realities exist.

When a doctor recognizes that a patient arrives not only with symptoms but also with concerns shaped by family, finances, and personal identity, the interaction changes subtly. The consultation becomes more than a technical process of diagnosing disease.

It becomes a human encounter within which medicine is practiced.

The chapters that follow explore this broader perspective—the understanding that patients are not merely biological cases, but individuals whose illnesses unfold within the complex landscape of their lives.

5.1 — Illness as a Personal Shock

For many patients, illness does not begin in the hospital or clinic. It begins quietly, often with a small change in the body that feels unusual or unfamiliar. A persistent headache, an unexplained pain, sudden fatigue, or a symptom that refuses to disappear can trigger a moment of concern.

At first, most people try to dismiss it.

They tell themselves it is temporary. Perhaps it is stress, lack of sleep, or something minor that will resolve on its own. Daily responsibilities continue—work, family obligations, routine tasks—and the symptom is pushed into the background of attention.

But when the discomfort persists, the mind begins to shift.

A subtle worry appears. The person begins to pay closer attention to the body. The same symptom that was ignored yesterday now becomes the subject of observation. Questions start forming silently.

Why is this happening? Why hasn't it improved yet?

This moment marks the beginning of a psychological transition.

The body, which normally functions without conscious awareness, suddenly becomes the center of attention. Every sensation feels significant. Minor changes are interpreted as signals that something may be wrong.

In many cases, the patient begins searching for explanations before meeting a doctor.

Conversations with friends or family may offer reassurance or sometimes amplify concern. Information found online can provide possible explanations but may also introduce alarming possibilities that increase anxiety. The mind begins to imagine outcomes that range from harmless to severe.

By the time the patient decides to consult a doctor, the emotional journey has already begun.

For some individuals, this journey includes days or weeks of silent worry. They may continue performing normal activities while privately questioning what the symptoms might mean. Work continues, social interactions continue, yet a quiet tension accompanies them.

This psychological tension often reaches its peak just before the medical consultation.

Walking into a clinic or hospital can feel like crossing an invisible threshold. On one side lies uncertainty and speculation. On the other lies the possibility of confirmation—either reassurance or a diagnosis that may change the course of life.

For the doctor, this consultation may appear routine. Another patient arrives, symptoms are described, and the process of diagnosis begins.

For the patient, however, the moment carries deeper significance.

They may be confronting the fear that something serious has developed inside their body. Even if the symptom appears minor from a clinical perspective, the patient's mind may already be exploring worst-case scenarios.

This emotional state shapes how the patient communicates with the doctor.

Some patients become very detailed in describing their symptoms, hoping that every piece of information will help the doctor understand the problem. Others become quiet or hesitant, unsure how to explain what they are feeling. In certain cases, fear may cause patients to exaggerate symptoms, while in other cases embarrassment may lead them to minimize them.

These reactions are not signs of irrational behavior. They reflect the human response to uncertainty about one's own health.

Illness introduces a sudden awareness of vulnerability. A person who felt physically normal days earlier now faces the possibility that something within the body may be malfunctioning.

Even before a diagnosis is made, this realization can be emotionally unsettling.

Understanding illness as a personal shock helps explain why patients sometimes appear anxious, impatient, or overly concerned about their symptoms. Their reactions are shaped not only by the physical condition itself but also by the psychological impact of confronting the unknown.

For doctors, recognizing this initial emotional state can transform the consultation experience.

The patient sitting across the table is not merely presenting symptoms. They are also arriving at the end of a private journey of worry, speculation, and hope that the doctor will provide clarity.

In this moment, medicine begins not only as a scientific investigation of disease, but also as a human response to uncertainty.

5.2— The Invisible Weight of Family Expectations

A patient rarely arrives at a clinic carrying only their own thoughts. Even when they walk into the consultation room alone, they often carry the voices, expectations, and concerns of many others.

Illness rarely affects only the individual who experiences it. It spreads quietly through families.

When someone begins to feel unwell, family members quickly become involved. A spouse may worry about how the illness will affect daily life. Parents may become anxious about their child's condition. Children may fear losing the stability that a healthy parent provides. Even extended family members sometimes participate in discussions about treatment and care.

The patient becomes the center of a collective concern.

In many cultures, particularly in societies where family bonds are strong, medical decisions are rarely made by the patient alone. A diagnosis may be discussed with parents, siblings, spouses, or elders before any major treatment is chosen. The doctor may see only one individual in the consultation room, but the decision-making process often involves many minds outside it.

This creates an invisible layer of pressure.

A patient may already be dealing with physical discomfort while also trying to manage the expectations of family members. Some relatives may urge immediate treatment. Others may recommend second opinions or alternative approaches. In some cases, family members express fear openly, increasing the patient's own anxiety.

Sometimes the pressure moves in the opposite direction.

A patient may feel responsible for protecting family members from worry. They may minimize their symptoms or avoid discussing their fears because they do not want to alarm their loved ones. A parent might continue working despite illness because they feel obligated to maintain stability for the family.

These emotional dynamics remain mostly hidden from the doctor.

In the consultation room, the patient may simply answer questions about symptoms and medical history. The doctor focuses on the biological aspects of the illness—what is happening in the body and how it should be treated.

Yet behind the patient's responses may lie a complex web of family expectations.

Consider a patient who hesitates when the doctor recommends hospitalization. The hesitation may not come from fear of the hospital itself but from concerns about family responsibilities. Who will care for children at home? Who will manage household responsibilities? How will the absence affect the family's daily routine?

These questions often remain unspoken during the consultation.

Family influence can also affect how patients interpret medical advice. Some relatives may encourage strict adherence to the doctor's recommendations, while others may question the treatment plan and suggest alternative options. In such situations, the patient may feel torn between trusting the doctor and responding to family opinions.

This internal conflict can make medical decisions emotionally difficult.

The doctor, observing the patient's uncertainty, may interpret hesitation as confusion or reluctance. In reality, the patient may be navigating a complex negotiation between medical advice and family expectations.

In certain cases, family pressure can even shape how symptoms are described.

A patient may exaggerate symptoms because family members insisted that the condition must be serious. Another patient may understate symptoms because they have been encouraged to remain strong and avoid appearing weak. Cultural beliefs about illness and responsibility often influence how individuals present their health concerns.

For the doctor, understanding these hidden dynamics is not always easy.

Time constraints and clinical focus often limit the depth of conversation during consultations. Yet recognizing that family expectations exist can help doctors interpret patient behavior more accurately.

When a patient appears hesitant, anxious, or indecisive, the reason may not lie solely in the illness itself.

It may lie in the invisible presence of the family standing quietly behind the patient's choices.

In this way, the consultation room becomes more than a meeting between doctor and patient. It becomes a moment where medicine intersects with family relationships, emotional responsibilities, and the complex social structures that shape human life.

5.3 — The Financial Reality of Illness

For many patients, illness is not experienced only as a medical problem. It is also a financial event. The moment a person realizes that treatment may be required, another set of questions quietly appears alongside the concern about health.

How much will this cost? Can I afford the treatment? What will happen if the expenses continue for months?

These questions may not always be spoken aloud during a consultation, but they often shape how patients approach medical care.

Medical treatment frequently involves multiple layers of expense. Diagnostic tests, specialist consultations, medications, hospital stays, and follow-up visits can accumulate quickly. Even when the disease itself is manageable, the financial impact of treatment may create additional stress for the patient and their family.

For individuals with stable financial resources or health insurance, these concerns may remain manageable. But for many people, especially in healthcare systems where patients bear significant portions of medical costs, the financial burden becomes a major factor in decision-making.

A patient may hesitate before agreeing to certain tests because they are calculating whether the cost will strain their household budget.

Sometimes patients delay seeking medical attention altogether. Symptoms that appear manageable are ignored for weeks or months because visiting a doctor might lead to expenses the family cannot easily bear. By the time the patient arrives at the clinic, the condition may have progressed beyond what early treatment could have addressed.

Financial stress therefore becomes intertwined with medical outcomes.

The doctor, focusing on clinical diagnosis, may recommend additional investigations or advanced treatment options based purely on medical reasoning. From a clinical perspective, these recommendations may represent the best path toward recovery.

But the patient may be evaluating the situation through a different lens.

Behind a simple response such as "I will think about it" may lie a complex financial calculation. The patient may be wondering whether they can afford the recommended test, whether they will need to borrow money, or whether treatment expenses might disrupt the family's financial stability.

In many cases, patients attempt to hide these concerns.

They may feel uncomfortable discussing financial limitations openly with the doctor. Some fear being judged or appearing incapable of following medical advice. Others may believe that doctors expect patients to prioritize treatment regardless of financial consequences.

As a result, the consultation sometimes proceeds without addressing the patient's economic reality.

This gap can lead to misunderstandings. A doctor may assume that a patient who does not follow recommended treatment is being careless or noncompliant. In reality, the patient may simply be unable to afford the proposed course of care.

The financial dimension of illness also affects emotional well-being.

Patients who worry about treatment costs may experience additional anxiety that compounds the stress of the disease itself. Instead of focusing solely on recovery, they must also consider how medical expenses will affect their household responsibilities, children's education, or long-term financial plans.

This pressure can be particularly intense for individuals who see themselves as primary providers for their families.

A person who becomes ill may not only worry about their own health but also about the economic consequences of being unable to work. Even a temporary illness can disrupt income, creating fear about how daily expenses will be managed.

In such situations, illness transforms from a medical challenge into a broader life crisis.

For doctors, understanding this dimension of patient experience does not mean abandoning medical judgment or compromising clinical standards. The physician's role remains centered on diagnosing and treating disease.

However, awareness of financial pressures can help doctors communicate more effectively.

When patients feel comfortable discussing economic concerns, doctors may be able to suggest alternative treatment plans, prioritize essential tests, or guide patients toward resources that reduce financial strain.

Recognizing the financial reality of illness reminds us that medicine does not operate in isolation from the economic structures of society.

A patient sitting in the consultation room may be confronting not only a biological condition but also a difficult financial decision—one that influences how they respond to medical advice and how they experience the journey toward recovery.

5.4 — Social Identity and Illness

Illness does not affect only the body. It also touches the roles a person holds in society. Every individual lives within a network of responsibilities and expectations—roles such as parent, provider, employee, student, or community member. When illness enters a person's life, these roles suddenly become uncertain.

For many patients, this uncertainty can be as troubling as the disease itself.

A person who is accustomed to being physically capable may struggle with the sudden realization that their body is no longer functioning as expected. Tasks that once felt effortless—working long hours, caring for children, or managing daily routines—may now require effort or may become temporarily impossible.

This shift challenges a person's sense of identity.

Consider someone who sees themselves primarily as the provider for their family. Illness may raise concerns about whether they can continue fulfilling that responsibility. A worker who supports household expenses may worry about missing workdays or losing income. Even a short period of illness can create anxiety about financial stability and professional reputation.

For parents, illness can introduce another layer of concern.

A mother or father who becomes sick may worry about how their children will react or who will manage household responsibilities during treatment. Even when the illness is manageable, the disruption to family life can weigh heavily on the patient's mind.

These concerns often remain unspoken during medical consultations.

The doctor may focus on diagnosing and treating the physical condition, while the patient is silently thinking about how the illness will affect their role in daily life. A diagnosis may therefore carry implications that extend far beyond the clinical setting.

Social perception also plays a role in how patients experience illness.

In some communities, certain diseases carry stigma or misunderstanding. Patients may fear being judged or treated differently by colleagues, neighbors, or relatives if their condition becomes known. This fear can lead individuals to delay seeking medical help or to hide symptoms from others.

The pressure to maintain social appearance can be powerful.

Some patients try to continue their normal routines despite worsening symptoms because they do not want others to perceive them as weak or incapable. They may postpone treatment until the illness becomes too serious to ignore.

For doctors, these social dynamics are not always visible.

A patient may appear calm and cooperative during the consultation, but internally they may be struggling with the thought of how the diagnosis will affect their work, family responsibilities, or social standing.

Even recommendations that seem straightforward from a medical perspective can create difficult decisions.

A doctor may advise rest for several weeks, but the patient may be thinking about job security. A hospital admission may be medically necessary, yet the patient may worry about leaving family members without support during that time.

These conflicts illustrate how illness intersects with the social structure of a person's life.

Medicine addresses the biological aspect of disease, but the patient experiences illness within the context of relationships, responsibilities, and identity. When these elements are disrupted, the emotional impact can be significant.

Understanding this dimension helps explain why patients sometimes respond to diagnoses with reactions that seem disproportionate to the medical condition itself.

What appears to be a manageable illness clinically may feel like a major disruption to the patient's life. The disease is not only affecting the body; it is reshaping the person's role within their social world.

Recognizing this reality allows doctors to see the consultation room differently.

The patient sitting across the table is not simply describing symptoms. They are also confronting questions about how their illness will affect who they are, what they do, and how they are perceived by the people around them.

In this sense, illness becomes more than a medical event—it becomes a moment where biology intersects with identity.

5.5 — Fear of the Unknown

For many patients, the most difficult part of illness is not always the disease itself but the uncertainty that surrounds it. The human mind tends to struggle more with the unknown than with confirmed reality. When a diagnosis has not yet been established, imagination often fills the gap.

This uncertainty begins the moment a person suspects that something may be wrong.

A persistent symptom, an unusual pain, or an unexpected change in the body can trigger a chain of thoughts that grows increasingly complex. At first, the person may hope the issue is minor. But as time passes and the symptom continues, uncertainty begins to expand.

The mind naturally searches for explanations.

In the absence of clear answers, people often turn to external sources for information. Conversations with friends, family members, or colleagues may introduce different interpretations of the symptom. Some may offer reassurance, while others may share stories that unintentionally increase anxiety.

In the modern world, the internet has become a powerful source of medical information.

Patients frequently search online for possible explanations of their symptoms before visiting a doctor. While access to medical knowledge can sometimes help patients understand their condition better, it can also expose them to alarming possibilities without proper context.

A mild symptom may suddenly appear linked to severe diseases through online searches.

This process can intensify fear even before the patient enters the clinic.

By the time the consultation takes place, the patient's mind may already be filled with imagined scenarios. Some may fear a life-threatening illness. Others may worry about long-term complications or permanent changes to their lifestyle. Even when the actual condition turns out to be relatively minor, the emotional stress experienced during the period of uncertainty can be significant.

Waiting for medical confirmation is often the most stressful stage.

When doctors recommend diagnostic tests, patients enter a new phase of waiting. Blood tests, imaging scans, or specialist evaluations may require several hours or days before results become available. During this time, the patient remains suspended between possibilities.

Every delay in receiving results may feel longer than it actually is.

In these moments, the patient's imagination often becomes the primary source of interpretation. Some people repeatedly review their symptoms in their minds, trying to identify patterns or signals that confirm or dismiss their fears. Others search for reassurance from family members or revisit online information.

This mental loop can be exhausting.

Even routine medical procedures can appear intimidating when viewed through the lens of uncertainty. A simple test recommended by the doctor may be interpreted by the patient as evidence that the problem might be serious.

The doctor, on the other hand, may see the test as a standard precaution.

This difference in perception sometimes leads to misunderstanding. The physician is following clinical reasoning—ordering tests to confirm or rule out possibilities. The patient, however, may interpret the same action as a signal that the situation is alarming.

Fear thrives in the absence of explanation.

When patients do not fully understand why certain tests are necessary or what the possible outcomes might be, their anxiety often increases. Even brief moments of clear communication from the doctor can help reduce this uncertainty.

Explaining that a test is routine or clarifying the range of possible diagnoses can restore a sense of stability.

Understanding the patient's fear of the unknown does not mean eliminating all uncertainty. Medicine itself often operates within probabilities rather than absolute certainty. Some conditions reveal their nature only through observation over time.

However, acknowledging the emotional impact of uncertainty can change the tone of medical interactions.

For patients, the period before a diagnosis is often filled with silent anxiety. Recognizing this emotional state allows doctors to respond not only as clinicians investigating disease but also as professionals guiding patients through the uncertain territory that illness creates.

In this way, medicine becomes not only a process of identifying biological conditions but also a way of helping individuals navigate the psychological space between fear and understanding.

5.6 — Communication Gaps Between Doctors and Patients

One of the most subtle challenges in medicine does not arise from biology or technology. It arises from communication. Doctors and patients often approach the same conversation from completely different perspectives, each shaped by their own experiences, expectations, and emotional states.

For the doctor, the consultation is a structured professional task.

The physician listens to symptoms, asks targeted questions, performs an examination, and begins constructing a clinical explanation for what may be happening in the patient's body. Medical training teaches doctors to filter information efficiently, focusing on details that are most relevant to diagnosis.

This approach is logical and necessary.

But the patient enters the consultation with a different mindset.

Patients rarely organize their experiences in the precise structure that medical training requires. Their descriptions may include emotions, personal experiences, and observations that feel important to them but may appear medically irrelevant. They may begin telling their story from the moment they first noticed the symptom, describing everything that happened along the way.

For the doctor, time constraints may require guiding the conversation toward specific details.

This difference in conversational style can create a subtle disconnect.

Doctors often speak the language of medicine—terms that reflect scientific understanding of the body. Words such as "inflammation," "benign," "chronic," or "prognosis" carry precise meanings in medical contexts. For physicians, these terms are part of everyday communication.

For patients, however, such language may feel unfamiliar or confusing.

Even when doctors try to simplify explanations, the patient may struggle to interpret the information correctly. A technical term intended to reassure may accidentally increase anxiety if the patient misunderstands its meaning.

Communication gaps can also arise from emotional differences.

Doctors approach illness with professional detachment developed through years of training. They have seen many conditions before and understand their typical progression. Patients, on the other hand, may be encountering the situation for the first time in their lives.

What appears routine to the doctor may feel alarming to the patient.

For example, a physician may calmly recommend additional tests as a standard diagnostic step. The patient may interpret the same recommendation as evidence that something serious is suspected.

This difference in interpretation can lead to confusion or fear.

Another source of communication difficulty is the limited time available for consultations. In busy healthcare environments, doctors often need to see many patients within a short period. This pressure can shorten conversations, leaving little space for patients to ask questions or express concerns.

When patients leave the consultation with unanswered questions, uncertainty can persist.

They may continue worrying about symptoms or misunderstand instructions for treatment. Sometimes patients hesitate to ask questions during the consultation because they feel the doctor is too busy.

These moments of hesitation can create gaps in understanding.

Communication also involves nonverbal signals. Tone of voice, facial expressions, and body language influence how messages are received. A doctor who appears rushed or distracted may unintentionally give the impression of disinterest, even if their clinical attention is focused on solving the problem.

Patients are highly sensitive to these signals.

A calm explanation or a brief moment of attentive listening can significantly change how patients perceive the interaction. When patients feel that the doctor has genuinely heard their concerns, trust grows naturally.

Closing the communication gap does not require long speeches or complex techniques.

Often it begins with simple clarity. Explaining medical terms in everyday language, briefly outlining why certain tests are needed, or asking patients whether they have questions can transform the consultation.

These small gestures remind patients that medicine is not only about diagnosing disease but also about guiding individuals through experiences that are unfamiliar and often frightening.

When communication becomes clearer, the consultation changes character. It becomes not merely a clinical exchange of information but a collaborative effort between doctor and patient to understand and address the problem together.

5.7 — Seeing the Whole Patient

Modern medicine is built upon extraordinary scientific knowledge. Doctors study anatomy, physiology, pathology, pharmacology, and countless other aspects of human biology in order to understand disease at its most detailed level. This scientific foundation allows physicians to diagnose illnesses, prescribe treatments, and perform procedures that can restore health and save lives.

Yet scientific knowledge alone does not fully capture the reality of the person sitting in the consultation room.

A patient arrives with more than a biological condition. They bring their fears about the future, their responsibilities toward family, their financial concerns, and their personal understanding of what illness means for their life. These elements may not appear in laboratory reports or imaging scans, but they shape how the patient experiences the disease.

Seeing the whole patient means recognizing this broader human context.

For a doctor, this awareness does not require abandoning scientific rigor. Diagnosis and treatment must remain grounded in medical evidence. The physician's responsibility is to understand what is happening in the body and to determine the most appropriate medical response.

However, when doctors remain aware that illness affects the entire life of the patient, their approach to care becomes more complete.

Two patients with the same diagnosis may respond very differently to treatment. One may follow medical advice carefully and recover smoothly. Another may struggle to follow the same treatment plan because of personal circumstances such as work pressure, family responsibilities, or financial limitations.

If the doctor sees only the disease, these differences may appear puzzling.

If the doctor sees the whole patient, the reasons become clearer.

Understanding the patient's situation helps doctors communicate more effectively. A physician who knows that a patient is worried about missing work may explain the importance of rest more carefully. A doctor who senses anxiety about a diagnosis may spend an extra moment clarifying what the condition means and what it does not mean.

These small adjustments can significantly influence how patients respond to medical care.

Seeing the whole patient also strengthens trust.

When patients feel that the doctor recognizes them as individuals rather than simply as cases, they become more comfortable sharing concerns. They may speak more openly about symptoms, fears, or practical challenges they are facing. This openness often improves the doctor's ability to make accurate clinical decisions.

The consultation then becomes a more complete exchange of information.

Doctors do not need to solve every problem in a patient's life. Their role remains focused on medical care. But acknowledging the human dimensions surrounding illness creates a more supportive environment in which treatment can succeed.

This perspective also reminds doctors that their profession occupies a unique position in society.

Few interactions are as intimate as the moment when someone discusses their health with a physician. Patients reveal physical discomfort, emotional worries, and personal circumstances that they may not share elsewhere. The doctor becomes a witness to these experiences while maintaining professional responsibility.

Seeing the whole patient therefore means recognizing the privilege and responsibility embedded in that position.

Medicine is not practiced only on the biological body. It is practiced within the lived reality of human beings whose health influences every aspect of their lives.

When doctors maintain this awareness, the practice of medicine becomes more than the management of disease.

It becomes an act of understanding—where science addresses the illness, and awareness acknowledges the human life that surrounds it.

Beyond the Diagnosis

At the end of a medical consultation, a diagnosis may be written, a prescription may be given, and the next steps in treatment may be explained. From a clinical perspective, this moment marks the completion of a medical task. The doctor has identified the problem and initiated the process of addressing it.

But for the patient, the experience rarely ends there.

The diagnosis becomes part of a much larger story unfolding in their life. After leaving the clinic, the patient carries the information back into their daily world—into conversations with family members, into decisions about work, into quiet moments of reflection about what the future might hold.

The illness becomes integrated into the patient's personal narrative.

Some diagnoses bring relief because they explain symptoms that were causing anxiety. Others introduce new uncertainties about treatment, recovery, or long-term health. Even conditions that are medically manageable can reshape how a person thinks about their body and their life.

In this way, the meaning of a diagnosis extends far beyond the medical record.

For doctors, understanding this broader impact helps illuminate the true complexity of their role. The physician does not simply identify diseases. They guide people through moments when biological changes intersect with emotional, social, and practical realities.

The consultation therefore becomes more than a technical interaction.

When a patient sits across from a doctor, they are seeking not only scientific expertise but also clarity during a moment of vulnerability. The doctor's explanation, tone, and attentiveness influence how the patient interprets the situation.

A calm and thoughtful conversation can transform fear into understanding. A rushed interaction can leave uncertainty lingering even when the medical advice is correct.

Recognizing the patient beyond biology does not mean that doctors must become counselors for every personal concern. The primary responsibility of the physician remains rooted in medical science and effective treatment.

However, acknowledging the human context of illness changes the atmosphere in which medicine is practiced.

It reminds doctors that each case represents a person navigating a complex life outside the clinic walls. It reminds patients that doctors, despite their clinical focus, are attempting to help them regain stability in that life.

When this awareness exists on both sides, the doctor–patient relationship becomes more balanced.

The doctor brings knowledge, training, and responsibility. The patient brings experience, vulnerability, and trust.

Between these two roles lies the true practice of medicine.

Diagnosis identifies the disease, but understanding the person transforms treatment into healing.

Chapter 6 — Medicine as a Participatory Field

Medicine Is Never a Two-Person Story

When people imagine medicine, they often picture a simple scene: a patient sitting across from a doctor. The patient explains symptoms, the doctor listens, examines, and prescribes treatment. This image has become the familiar symbol of healthcare—a private conversation between two individuals focused on solving a biological problem.

Yet the reality of medicine is far more complex.

What appears to be a two-person interaction is actually the visible surface of a much larger system. The consultation room may contain only a doctor and a patient, but behind them stand many other participants whose influence shapes what happens in that moment.

A patient rarely arrives alone in a meaningful sense.

Even if they enter the clinic without family members present, they carry the concerns and expectations of those close to them. Their spouse may have encouraged the visit. Their parents may be waiting for updates. Their children may depend on the outcome of the treatment. Financial responsibilities, social roles, and family relationships quietly accompany the patient into the consultation.

On the other side of the table, the doctor is not acting entirely as an independent professional.

The physician operates within a structured system that includes hospitals, clinics, administrative policies, medical guidelines, and professional regulations. The doctor's decisions are shaped not only by knowledge and experience but also by the resources available within that system.

A recommendation for treatment may depend on what facilities the hospital provides, what medications are accessible, or what protocols the institution follows.

Beyond the immediate environment of the hospital lies an even wider circle of influence.

Healthcare systems exist within societies that carry expectations about how medicine should function. Patients expect compassion, accuracy, and affordability. Governments establish regulations to ensure safety and accountability. Media coverage influences public perception of doctors and hospitals.

These broader forces quietly influence the interactions that occur inside the consultation room.

When a doctor recommends a test, that decision is supported by laboratory technicians who will perform the analysis. When a patient receives medication, pharmacists and manufacturers become part of the chain that delivers treatment. Nurses, administrative staff, and healthcare workers coordinate countless tasks that make the system function.

Medicine therefore operates less like a simple transaction and more like a living network.

Each participant contributes something essential. The doctor provides knowledge and clinical judgment. The patient provides information about symptoms and follows treatment plans. Families offer support or sometimes pressure. Institutions provide infrastructure and coordination. Society establishes expectations and regulations.

Health outcomes emerge from the interaction of all these elements.

When this network functions smoothly, treatment appears straightforward. The doctor diagnoses the condition, the patient follows the advice, and recovery progresses as expected. But when tensions arise within this network—miscommunication, distrust, institutional limitations—the entire process becomes more complicated.

Understanding medicine as a participatory field reveals an important truth.

Healing is rarely produced by the actions of a single individual. It emerges from the cooperation of many participants whose roles intersect in ways that are often invisible.

The chapters that follow explore this wider field of participation. Because to understand modern medicine fully, we must look beyond the consultation table and recognize the complex web of relationships that surrounds every act of care.

6.1 — The Consultation Is Only the Surface

When a patient enters a clinic and sits across from a doctor, the scene appears simple. Two individuals face each other, discussing symptoms and possible treatments. The doctor asks questions, listens carefully, examines the patient, and eventually offers a diagnosis or recommendation.

To an outside observer, this interaction may seem like the entire process of medicine.

But in reality, the consultation is only the visible surface of a much larger structure. It is the point where many invisible influences converge into a single moment of decision.

Behind every medical consultation lies a network of factors that shape what happens inside the room.

Consider the patient's journey before arriving at the clinic. The decision to seek medical help rarely happens instantly. The patient may have spent days or weeks observing symptoms, discussing concerns with family members, searching for information, or debating whether the problem is serious enough to require professional attention.

By the time the patient meets the doctor, these thoughts and conversations have already shaped expectations and emotions.

Similarly, the doctor does not enter the consultation as a completely independent decision-maker. The physician's medical training, hospital guidelines, available diagnostic tools, and institutional protocols all influence how the consultation unfolds.

For example, a doctor may suspect a particular condition but must confirm it through tests available within the hospital's laboratory system. The decision to recommend certain treatments may depend on what medications are accessible or what procedures the institution is equipped to perform.

The consultation room therefore functions as a node where many unseen systems intersect.

Even the physical setting reflects this complexity. The patient sits in a hospital or clinic built through organizational planning, managed by administrative staff, supported by nurses and technicians, and regulated by healthcare policies. The doctor's knowledge itself is the result of years of education shaped by universities, medical boards, and scientific research.

All of these elements silently influence the interaction.

When the doctor listens to symptoms and begins forming a diagnosis, they are drawing not only from personal experience but also from the collective knowledge of medical science. When the patient describes discomfort or anxiety, those expressions are shaped by personal circumstances, cultural beliefs, and family influence.

Thus, the consultation becomes more than a conversation.

It becomes the moment where two complex systems meet: the personal world of the patient and the professional world of medicine.

The patient represents a life filled with responsibilities, relationships, fears, and expectations. The doctor represents a profession guided by scientific knowledge, institutional structures, and ethical responsibilities.

Inside the consultation room, these two worlds attempt to understand each other.

The doctor tries to interpret symptoms within a biological framework. The patient tries to interpret the doctor's words within the context of their life situation.

When communication flows clearly, this interaction works smoothly. The doctor gathers accurate information, the patient understands the treatment plan, and the healthcare system supports the process with appropriate resources.

But when misunderstandings arise, the consultation reveals how fragile this surface interaction can be.

A patient may misunderstand medical instructions because the explanation was too technical. A doctor may assume that a treatment plan will be followed without realizing that financial or family pressures make it difficult.

In such moments, the consultation room becomes a place where deeper tensions within the healthcare system begin to appear.

Recognizing that the consultation is only the surface helps us see medicine differently. What appears to be a simple interaction between doctor and patient is actually the visible point where multiple layers of participation—personal, professional, institutional, and social—come together.

Understanding this deeper structure allows us to see why healthcare outcomes depend not only on medical knowledge but also on how effectively this entire network of participants works together.

6.2 — The Patient's Network of Influence

When a patient enters the consultation room, it may appear that the individual is making decisions independently. The doctor asks questions, the patient answers, and together they discuss possible treatments. From a clinical perspective, this interaction seems direct and straightforward.

Yet the patient rarely represents only their own perspective.

Behind every patient stands a network of relationships and influences that shape how medical decisions are understood and accepted. Family members, cultural beliefs, social expectations, and past experiences with healthcare all quietly influence the choices that the patient makes.

This network may not always be visible during the consultation, but it plays a powerful role in shaping outcomes.

Family is often the most immediate influence.

In many households, illness becomes a shared concern rather than a private matter. When someone begins experiencing symptoms, relatives quickly become involved in the discussion. Advice is offered, worries are expressed, and opinions about possible treatments begin to circulate.

By the time the patient meets the doctor, these conversations may already have shaped expectations.

A family member may have insisted that the patient see a doctor immediately. Another may have suggested waiting longer to see if the condition improves. Someone else may have shared stories about similar symptoms and their own experiences with treatment.

These influences affect how the patient interprets the doctor's advice.

For example, a doctor may recommend a particular medication or procedure based on medical reasoning. The patient, however, may consider how family members will react to that recommendation.

Will relatives support the treatment? Will they worry about side effects? Will they suggest alternative approaches?

The patient's response may therefore reflect not only personal judgment but also the anticipated reaction of others.

Cultural beliefs also play an important role.

Different societies carry distinct understandings of health, illness, and healing. Some communities place strong trust in modern medical science, while others combine medical treatment with traditional practices or spiritual interpretations of illness.

Patients often bring these beliefs with them into the consultation.

A doctor may describe a disease using scientific language and recommend a clear treatment plan. The patient may interpret that explanation through cultural ideas about the body, balance, or natural remedies. Sometimes these perspectives align smoothly; other times they create uncertainty.

Social expectations add another layer of influence.

In many cultures, individuals feel pressure to appear strong and resilient, especially when they hold important roles within the family or workplace. As a result, some patients minimize their symptoms or delay treatment because they do not want to appear weak or incapable.

Others may feel pressure from family members to pursue aggressive treatment even when they personally feel uncertain.

Past experiences with healthcare systems also shape patient attitudes.

Someone who has previously received effective care may approach the doctor with trust and openness. Another person who has experienced long waiting times, financial difficulties, or negative encounters may approach the consultation with caution or skepticism.

These past experiences influence how patients interpret the doctor's recommendations.

For the physician, understanding this network of influence can be challenging because many of these factors remain unspoken. The consultation often focuses on medical information, leaving little time to explore the broader context surrounding the patient's decisions.

Yet recognizing that this network exists can help doctors interpret patient behavior more accurately.

When a patient hesitates before agreeing to treatment, the reason may not be medical confusion. It may be the result of discussions that will take place later with family members. When a patient asks repeated questions about a diagnosis, they may be preparing to explain the situation to relatives who will also participate in the decision.

Seen in this light, the patient is not simply an isolated individual making medical choices.

They are a participant within a larger web of relationships and beliefs that shape how illness is understood and how treatment is accepted.

In the participatory field of medicine, this network becomes one of the most important influences guiding what ultimately happens after the consultation ends.

6.3 — The Doctor Inside a System

Patients often imagine the doctor as a completely independent decision-maker—someone who examines symptoms, determines the diagnosis, and chooses the best possible treatment based purely on medical knowledge. In this view, the doctor stands at the center of the healing process, exercising authority and expertise without limitation.

In reality, the doctor operates within a much larger structure.

Modern medicine functions through institutions—hospitals, clinics, laboratories, regulatory bodies, and healthcare systems that organize how care is delivered. The doctor's role exists within this framework rather than outside it. Every consultation and treatment decision is influenced, directly or indirectly, by the systems that surround the physician.

The hospital itself is one of the most immediate influences.

Hospitals operate through policies and protocols designed to ensure patient safety and consistency of care. Clinical guidelines outline recommended treatments for many conditions. Standard procedures govern how tests are ordered, how medications are prescribed, and how patient records are maintained.

These structures help maintain quality and accountability in healthcare.

However, they also shape the way doctors practice medicine. A physician may recognize several possible approaches to treating a condition, but the final choice often depends on what resources are available within the institution.

For example, certain diagnostic technologies may exist in one hospital but not in another. Some medications may be readily available, while others may require special approval. Surgical procedures may depend on the presence of specialized teams or equipment.

Thus, medical decisions are not made in a vacuum.

Time constraints also influence how doctors interact with patients. In busy healthcare systems, physicians may be responsible for seeing many patients within limited hours. Clinics must maintain schedules, emergency departments must manage continuous inflow, and hospitals must coordinate care across multiple departments.

As a result, doctors often work within tightly structured time frames.

This reality can create tension between the ideal of unlimited patient attention and the practical demands of the healthcare system. A physician may wish to spend more time discussing a patient's concerns, but the schedule may require moving quickly to the next consultation.

Administrative responsibilities add another layer to the doctor's work.

Modern healthcare involves extensive documentation. Doctors must record diagnoses, treatment plans, test results, and clinical observations in patient records. These records serve many purposes—they guide future treatment, ensure continuity of care, and meet legal and regulatory requirements.

While documentation improves accountability, it also consumes a significant portion of a doctor's time.

Many physicians find themselves balancing clinical duties with administrative tasks, reviewing reports, completing digital records, and communicating with other healthcare professionals involved in patient care.

In addition to institutional responsibilities, doctors must also follow professional regulations.

Medical boards, licensing authorities, and healthcare regulations establish standards for safe and ethical practice. Doctors must remain aware of these rules when making decisions about treatment, prescriptions, and procedures.

This regulatory environment protects patients but also adds another layer of responsibility to the physician's role.

Within this complex system, the doctor becomes both a decision-maker and a participant.

The physician applies medical knowledge and clinical judgment, but those decisions are shaped by the structures that enable healthcare to function. Nurses, technicians, pharmacists, and administrative staff all contribute to the delivery of treatment.

Laboratories process tests, imaging departments provide diagnostic information, and support staff coordinate appointments and patient flow.

Medicine therefore operates as a coordinated system rather than an individual effort.

Recognizing the doctor as part of this system helps explain why medical care sometimes feels constrained by factors beyond the doctor's control. Delays in test results, limited resources, or institutional policies may influence the pace and direction of treatment.

For patients, understanding this reality can provide a more complete picture of how healthcare works.

The doctor remains central to the process, but the effectiveness of medical care depends on the broader system that supports the physician's work. Within the participatory field of medicine, the doctor is not an isolated authority but a key participant operating within an intricate network designed to sustain health and healing.

6.4 — Hospitals as Complex Organisms

When patients think about healthcare, they often imagine hospitals as places where doctors diagnose diseases and prescribe treatments. From the outside, a hospital may appear to be a single institution with clear roles and straightforward processes. Yet inside, a hospital functions more like a complex organism—an interconnected system in which many parts must work together continuously.

No single individual delivers healthcare alone.

While the doctor often becomes the visible face of treatment, the functioning of a hospital depends on a wide network of professionals who coordinate their efforts behind the scenes. Nurses monitor patients, administer medications, and observe changes in condition. Laboratory technicians analyze blood and tissue samples. Radiology teams operate imaging equipment that reveals internal structures of the body.

Each of these roles contributes essential information to the doctor's decision-making process.

Consider what happens when a physician orders a diagnostic test. The request moves through several layers of the hospital system. A technician performs the test, laboratory specialists analyze the results, digital systems record the findings, and finally the doctor reviews the report before deciding on the next step in treatment.

What appears to be a simple instruction from the doctor is actually the beginning of a coordinated chain of activity.

Hospitals also depend on professionals whose work remains largely invisible to patients. Pharmacists manage medication supplies and verify prescriptions. Biomedical engineers maintain medical equipment. Administrative staff organize patient records, appointments, and insurance documentation.

Even the cleanliness and safety of hospital environments depend on support staff who ensure that infection control standards are maintained.

These coordinated efforts allow the healthcare system to function reliably.

When this coordination works smoothly, the patient experiences care as a continuous and organized process. Tests are completed, results are delivered, medications are administered, and recovery progresses through structured stages.

But when coordination breaks down, the effects quickly become visible.

Delays in communication between departments may postpone diagnosis. A shortage of staff may slow patient care. Miscommunication between professionals may create confusion about treatment plans. In such situations, patients sometimes assume that the doctor alone is responsible for the difficulty.

In reality, the challenge often lies within the broader system.

Hospitals must manage thousands of interactions every day. Emergency cases arrive unexpectedly. Intensive care units require constant monitoring. Surgical teams coordinate complex procedures involving multiple specialists.

The hospital therefore operates as a dynamic environment where many processes occur simultaneously.

Within this environment, the doctor acts as a central participant but not the only one. The physician interprets medical information and guides treatment decisions, yet these decisions rely heavily on the coordinated work of the entire hospital team.

This is why communication within hospitals is so critical.

Doctors must exchange information with nurses, technicians, and other specialists to ensure that treatment proceeds accurately. A small detail observed by a nurse during patient monitoring may provide crucial information for the physician's next decision. Similarly, laboratory findings may reveal patterns that shape the entire treatment plan.

Seen from this perspective, the hospital resembles a living organism.

Just as the organs of the human body must function together to maintain health, the different departments of a hospital must coordinate effectively to sustain patient care. Each component contributes something essential, and the failure of one part can affect the whole system.

For patients, understanding this complexity can change how the hospital experience is perceived.

The doctor remains a central guide in the process of treatment, but the success of medical care depends on the cooperation of an entire network of professionals working together within the hospital environment.

In the participatory field of medicine, the hospital becomes not merely a building where treatment occurs, but a dynamic system through which knowledge, technology, and human effort converge to support healing.

6.5 — Society's Expectations of Medicine

Medicine does not exist only within hospitals and clinics. It also lives within the expectations of society. Every community carries certain beliefs about what doctors should do, how healthcare should function, and what outcomes should be expected from medical treatment.

These expectations shape the environment in which doctors practice.

For many people, doctors represent the highest level of authority in matters of health. When someone becomes ill, the natural response is to seek professional help with the hope that the doctor will identify the problem and provide a solution. Over generations, medical science has made remarkable progress—curing infections, performing complex surgeries, and extending human life through advanced treatments.

These achievements have strengthened public confidence in medicine.

At the same time, they have also created powerful expectations.

Patients often approach healthcare with the belief that modern medicine should be able to fix most problems quickly and effectively. When treatment succeeds, this belief is reinforced. But when outcomes are uncertain or recovery takes longer than expected, frustration can arise.

Society sometimes forgets that medicine still operates within the limits of human knowledge and biological complexity.

Not every disease can be cured immediately. Some conditions require long-term management rather than complete elimination. Others remain unpredictable despite careful treatment.

Yet the public image of medicine often emphasizes success stories—dramatic recoveries, technological breakthroughs, and life-saving interventions.

Media coverage plays an important role in shaping this perception.

Television programs, news reports, and social media often highlight extraordinary cases where doctors perform remarkable procedures or achieve impressive results. While these stories celebrate medical progress, they can also create unrealistic expectations about what healthcare can deliver in everyday situations.

Patients may arrive at hospitals expecting quick answers and guaranteed solutions.

Doctors, however, must work within the realities of biology, available resources, and individual patient conditions. This difference between expectation and reality sometimes creates tension in the doctor–patient relationship.

Society also expects doctors to embody certain ethical standards.

Physicians are expected to be knowledgeable, responsible, and compassionate. People often assume that doctors should place patient welfare above all other considerations. This expectation reflects the deep trust that society places in medical professionals.

At the same time, doctors themselves are part of the same social environment.

They face financial pressures, institutional constraints, and personal responsibilities like anyone else. Balancing professional dedication with practical realities can sometimes be challenging.

Public discussions about healthcare often focus on the responsibilities of doctors while paying less attention to the broader system in which they work.

For example, healthcare infrastructure, government policies, insurance systems, and hospital management all influence how care is delivered. Yet when problems arise, the doctor frequently becomes the most visible figure to whom frustration is directed.

This dynamic illustrates how society participates in the field of medicine.

Patients bring expectations about healing, fairness, and affordability. Governments establish regulations to protect public health. Media narratives influence public perception of doctors and hospitals.

Together, these forces create the social environment in which medical practice unfolds.

For doctors, navigating these expectations requires not only clinical skill but also awareness of how society interprets their role. Patients often arrive with hopes shaped by cultural beliefs, family experiences, and public narratives about medicine.

Understanding these expectations can help doctors communicate more effectively.

When physicians explain the limits as well as the possibilities of medical treatment, they help align patient expectations with reality. Honest communication can transform frustration into understanding and strengthen trust within the healthcare system.

In this way, society becomes an active participant in the medical field.

The relationship between doctors and patients is influenced not only by clinical decisions but also by the collective beliefs and expectations that communities hold about health, illness, and healing.

6.6 — When Participation Breaks Down

When all the participants in healthcare work in alignment—doctors, patients, families, hospitals, and society—the process of treatment often feels smooth and cooperative. The patient explains symptoms honestly, the doctor evaluates them carefully, the hospital system supports diagnosis and treatment, and families provide encouragement and practical support.

In such situations, medicine functions as a coordinated effort.

But the participatory nature of healthcare also means that when one part of the system fails to align with the others, the entire process can become strained. Conflicts begin to appear, misunderstandings grow, and trust between participants can weaken.

These breakdowns rarely occur because of a single cause.

Often they arise from small gaps in understanding that gradually widen. A patient may feel that the doctor did not listen carefully enough. The doctor may feel that the patient ignored important medical advice. Family members may question the treatment plan, and hospital staff may struggle to manage limited resources.

Each participant may believe they are acting responsibly, yet the system begins to lose harmony.

One common source of breakdown occurs through communication gaps.

Doctors may explain a diagnosis using clinical language that feels clear to them but confusing to the patient. The patient may leave the consultation uncertain about what was said but hesitate to ask further questions. Family members may later interpret the situation differently, creating additional confusion.

In this way, a simple misunderstanding can grow into mistrust.

Institutional pressures can also contribute to these breakdowns.

Hospitals must manage large numbers of patients, limited staff, and administrative requirements. Doctors may be forced to work within tight schedules that reduce the time available for detailed conversations. Patients, however, often arrive expecting personal attention and clear explanations.

When these expectations collide with the realities of busy healthcare systems, frustration can arise on both sides.

Financial pressures sometimes add further tension.

A patient who struggles to afford treatment may feel that the healthcare system prioritizes costs over care. Doctors, on the other hand, may feel frustrated when recommended treatments are delayed or refused because of financial concerns.

Both perspectives reflect genuine difficulties, yet they can lead to misunderstanding if not addressed openly.

Public perception also plays a role when participation breaks down.

Stories about medical errors or negative experiences spread quickly through communities and media channels. Even when such cases are rare, they can influence how patients approach future medical interactions. Suspicion or anxiety may replace the trust that once guided doctor–patient relationships.

Doctors, sensing this shift, may become more cautious or defensive in their interactions.

This cycle can gradually erode the cooperative spirit that medicine depends upon.

In extreme situations, the breakdown of participation can lead to open conflict—arguments between families and healthcare staff, accusations against doctors, or even legal disputes. When these events occur, they often attract public attention, reinforcing the perception that the healthcare system is failing.

Yet beneath these visible conflicts lies a deeper issue.

Medicine functions best when its participants recognize their shared purpose: restoring health and stability to human lives. When each participant begins to see the others as adversaries rather than partners, the system loses the collaborative energy that allows it to function effectively.

Understanding this dynamic is essential.

Doctors must recognize the fears and expectations that patients bring into the consultation. Patients must recognize the pressures and limitations under which doctors operate. Institutions must provide environments that support clear communication and fair access to care.

When these elements align again, trust begins to rebuild.

The participatory field of medicine therefore reminds us that healthcare is not sustained by knowledge alone. It depends equally on cooperation, understanding, and the willingness of all participants to recognize their role in maintaining the delicate balance that allows healing to occur.

6.7 — Seeing Healthcare as a Field, Not a Transaction

Modern healthcare is often described in transactional terms. A patient visits a doctor, a consultation takes place, treatment is prescribed, and the interaction ends. From this perspective, medicine can appear similar to a service exchange—one person seeking help and another providing expertise.

But this view captures only a small part of what actually happens.

Healthcare does not function as a simple transaction. It operates more like a field of participation in which multiple individuals and systems interact continuously. The doctor, the patient, the family, the hospital, and society all contribute to the outcome of medical care.

Each participant influences the process in ways that may not always be visible.

The doctor brings knowledge, clinical judgment, and professional responsibility. Years of training allow the physician to interpret symptoms and design treatment strategies. But knowledge alone cannot guarantee recovery if the patient is unable to follow the treatment plan.

The patient, therefore, becomes an active participant rather than a passive recipient of care.

Recovery often depends on how carefully the patient follows medical advice, takes prescribed medication, attends follow-up appointments, and communicates changes in symptoms. The patient's attitude toward treatment—whether cooperative, hesitant, or skeptical—can significantly influence outcomes.

Family members also participate in this field.

They may provide emotional support that encourages the patient to follow treatment. They may assist with practical needs such as transportation to hospitals or assistance during recovery. In some cases, family members influence decisions about whether treatment should begin, continue, or change.

The hospital environment forms another layer of participation.

Doctors rely on nurses, technicians, pharmacists, and administrative staff to carry out the many tasks required for patient care. Diagnostic equipment, laboratory systems, and hospital infrastructure all contribute to the accuracy and efficiency of medical treatment.

Even society participates in shaping the healthcare field.

Public policies determine how healthcare systems are funded and regulated. Cultural beliefs influence how people perceive illness and treatment. Social trust affects how patients approach doctors and how doctors interact with the public.

Seen in this way, healthcare resembles a dynamic field rather than a sequence of isolated actions.

In a field, every participant influences the others. The doctor's communication affects patient confidence. The patient's cooperation affects treatment success. The hospital's efficiency affects the speed and quality of care. Social attitudes influence how the entire system is perceived.

When these elements align, the field becomes stable.

Doctors and patients work together with mutual understanding. Institutions support treatment effectively. Families provide encouragement rather than confusion. Society maintains trust in the medical profession.

In such an environment, healing becomes more likely.

But when participants view healthcare as a transaction, the field becomes fragmented.

Patients may see doctors only as service providers responsible for solving every problem. Doctors may view patients as cases that must be processed quickly within institutional constraints. Hospitals may focus primarily on efficiency, while society may judge outcomes without understanding the complexity behind them.

This fragmented view weakens cooperation.

Restoring the idea of healthcare as a participatory field helps rebuild balance.

It reminds doctors that treatment succeeds not only through medical knowledge but also through communication and trust. It reminds patients that recovery involves their own participation and responsibility. It reminds institutions and society that healthcare functions best when all participants support the process.

In this field, healing becomes a collective effort.

Medicine is no longer simply something done *to* a patient by a doctor. It becomes something created *between* many participants who together shape the conditions in which recovery can occur.

Healing as a Collective Process

When we look at medicine from a distance, it is easy to imagine healing as the result of a doctor's expertise. A patient becomes ill, a doctor identifies the problem, treatment is given, and recovery follows. This image places the doctor at the center of the process, as if healing flows primarily from the knowledge and skill of a single professional.

But the deeper reality of healthcare reveals something different.

Healing is rarely the work of one individual. It emerges from the combined participation of many people and systems working together. The doctor provides knowledge and clinical judgment. The patient brings trust, honesty, and commitment to treatment. Families offer support and care during moments of vulnerability.

Hospitals provide the infrastructure, staff, and technology necessary for diagnosis and treatment.

Beyond these immediate participants lies the wider society that shapes how healthcare operates. Public policies determine access to medical services. Cultural beliefs influence how people understand illness. Communities create the environment of trust—or distrust—within which medical relationships unfold.

All of these elements contribute to the process we call healing.

When this collective participation functions harmoniously, medicine becomes remarkably powerful. A patient feels confident sharing symptoms openly. The doctor listens carefully and applies scientific knowledge. Families cooperate with treatment plans. Hospitals coordinate their resources effectively.

In such an environment, the entire system works toward the same goal.

Yet when this participation becomes fragmented, medicine struggles.

Patients may doubt the intentions of doctors. Doctors may feel constrained by institutional pressures. Families may question treatment decisions. Society may view healthcare through suspicion rather than trust.

The field of participation becomes unstable.

Understanding healing as a collective process helps shift the way we think about responsibility in healthcare. Instead of asking who alone is responsible for success or failure, we begin to recognize that outcomes emerge from the interaction of many participants.

Doctors carry a unique responsibility because of their expertise and authority. But patients, families, institutions, and society also shape the environment in which healing occurs.

Each participant contributes something essential.

The patient contributes honesty about symptoms and commitment to recovery. The doctor contributes knowledge, judgment, and professional care. The family contributes emotional and practical support. The hospital contributes coordination and resources. Society contributes trust and structure.

When these contributions align, the process of healing becomes stronger than the effort of any single individual.

Seen in this light, medicine is not simply a service provided by doctors to patients. It is a collaborative effort unfolding within a complex human system.

The consultation room may appear to contain only two people, but the forces shaping that moment extend far beyond those walls.

Recognizing this shared participation helps restore balance to the understanding of healthcare.

Because healing, at its deepest level, is not only a medical act—it is a collective human endeavor where knowledge, trust, responsibility, and cooperation meet in the fragile yet hopeful space between illness and recovery.

Chapter 7 — The Doctor as a Stabilizing Node

The Quiet Center of the System

Within the complex field of healthcare, many participants contribute to the process of healing. Patients bring their symptoms and concerns. Families provide emotional support and practical assistance. Hospitals supply infrastructure, technology, and coordinated teams of professionals. Society establishes expectations about how medicine should function.

Yet within this network of participation, one figure often becomes the central point of stability—the doctor.

When illness enters a person's life, uncertainty quickly follows. Symptoms create questions that the patient cannot answer alone. Families become anxious about possible outcomes. Medical information may appear overwhelming or confusing. In these moments, the healthcare system may seem vast and complicated.

The doctor becomes the person who helps bring clarity to this uncertainty.

Patients look toward physicians not only for medical knowledge but also for direction. A diagnosis organizes scattered symptoms into a meaningful explanation. A treatment plan transforms anxiety into action. Even a simple reassurance that a condition is manageable can reduce the emotional weight that patients and families carry.

In this way, the doctor often becomes the point around which confusion begins to settle.

This stabilizing role extends beyond the consultation itself. When families discuss treatment options, the doctor's opinion often becomes the reference point for decision-making. When hospitals coordinate care between departments, physicians frequently guide the process through clinical leadership.

Even when technology and teams are involved, the doctor remains the figure who interprets information and provides direction.

The stability created by this role is not based solely on authority.

It arises from the trust that society has placed in the medical profession. People believe that doctors possess knowledge gained through years of training and that this knowledge is used responsibly to protect human life and well-being.

This trust gives the doctor's words significant weight.

A calm explanation from a physician can reduce fear. A clear recommendation can help families move forward with difficult decisions. In situations where uncertainty cannot be eliminated, the doctor's presence can still provide reassurance that the situation is being handled with care and competence.

However, this stabilizing influence also carries a quiet burden.

Doctors must often deliver guidance in moments when complete certainty is impossible. Medicine operates within probabilities rather than absolute guarantees. A physician may recommend treatment based on the best available evidence while still knowing that outcomes can vary.

Despite this uncertainty, patients continue to look toward the doctor for stability.

The physician therefore stands at a unique intersection within the healthcare system—between knowledge and uncertainty, between institutional systems and human emotion. The doctor becomes the point where scientific understanding meets the lived reality of illness.

In this position, the doctor functions not only as a provider of treatment but also as a stabilizing node within the entire healthcare field.

The chapters that follow explore how this role emerged, why society places such trust in physicians, and how the stability created by this trust shapes the functioning of the healthcare system itself.

7.1 — Why Society Trusts Doctors

The position that doctors hold in society did not emerge suddenly. It developed gradually over centuries as human communities searched for individuals who could understand illness and help restore health. In earlier times, healers relied on observation, experience, and traditional knowledge to treat the sick. These early practitioners were often respected because they possessed rare insight into the mysteries of the human body.

As medical science evolved, this respect began to transform into a deeper form of trust.

The development of anatomy, physiology, microbiology, and pharmacology allowed physicians to understand disease in ways that were previously impossible. Scientific discoveries revealed how infections spread, how organs function, and how medicines interact with the body. Treatments became more effective and predictable.

Each advancement strengthened society's confidence in the medical profession.

Hospitals improved survival rates for serious illnesses. Vaccinations protected populations from dangerous diseases. Surgical techniques restored health where previously there had been little hope. Over time, people began to associate doctors with the power of scientific knowledge and the ability to intervene meaningfully in human suffering.

This connection between science and care created a powerful foundation for trust.

Unlike many professions, medicine deals directly with the most vulnerable moments of human life. When people fall ill, they must reveal personal details about their bodies, their habits, and their fears. Patients allow doctors to examine them physically and to make decisions that may affect their future health.

Such openness requires confidence in the integrity of the physician.

For this reason, medical education has always emphasized ethical responsibility alongside scientific training. Doctors are taught that their knowledge must be used for the benefit of patients and not for personal gain. Professional codes of conduct, such as the long-standing principles of medical ethics, reinforce the idea that physicians carry a special duty toward those who seek their help.

These ethical expectations reinforce society's willingness to trust doctors.

The public believes that physicians are guided not only by knowledge but also by responsibility. When patients follow medical advice, they are placing their well-being in the hands of someone they believe is committed to protecting it.

Trust is therefore built on two foundations: competence and integrity.

Competence assures patients that the doctor understands the science of medicine. Integrity assures them that this knowledge will be used with care and honesty.

This combination places doctors in a unique position within society.

Few other professions require such deep levels of trust. Patients often meet doctors during moments when they feel physically weak or emotionally vulnerable. In these moments, they rely on the physician's judgment without fully understanding the medical reasoning behind it.

The doctor becomes a guide through unfamiliar territory.

This trust extends beyond individual interactions. Communities often look to doctors as reliable sources of information about health risks, disease prevention, and medical decisions that affect public well-being. During outbreaks of disease or public health crises, physicians frequently become important voices guiding society through uncertainty.

Yet the trust placed in doctors also brings expectations.

Society expects physicians to maintain high standards of professionalism, to communicate honestly, and to treat patients with fairness and respect. When doctors meet these expectations, trust grows stronger. When failures occur—whether through negligence, miscommunication, or systemic pressures—public confidence can be shaken.

Understanding why society trusts doctors helps explain the stabilizing role that physicians play within healthcare.

Because when people believe that a doctor is knowledgeable, ethical, and committed to their well-being, the doctor's presence alone can help restore a sense of order in situations where illness has created uncertainty.

7.2 — The Doctor as a Point of Decision

Within the healthcare system, many participants contribute to the process of treatment. Patients describe symptoms, families provide support, nurses monitor daily changes, technicians conduct diagnostic tests, and hospitals coordinate the infrastructure required for care. Each participant plays an important role.

Yet when uncertainty reaches a critical point, the responsibility for decision often converges on the doctor.

Medicine frequently involves situations where multiple possibilities must be considered at the same time. Symptoms may point toward several different conditions. Diagnostic tests may provide clues but not always complete certainty. Treatment options may involve different risks and benefits.

In these moments, someone must decide how to proceed.

The doctor becomes that point of decision.

This responsibility arises because physicians are trained to interpret complex medical information and evaluate probabilities. Years of study and clinical experience teach doctors how to recognize patterns in symptoms, understand the mechanisms of disease, and anticipate how different treatments may influence the body.

This knowledge allows doctors to make informed judgments when situations remain uncertain.

Consider a patient presenting with chest pain. The symptom could indicate something minor, such as muscle strain, or something serious, such as a heart condition. Diagnostic tests provide valuable information, but they may not always deliver immediate or definitive answers.

The doctor must decide which tests to perform, how urgently they are needed, and whether treatment should begin immediately.

In such situations, delay itself can become a risk.

The physician must weigh the available evidence and choose a course of action that balances caution with urgency. These decisions often occur quickly, especially in emergency settings where time is limited and the patient's condition may change rapidly.

Families and patients often look to the doctor for guidance in these moments.

When faced with multiple treatment options, patients may feel overwhelmed by the complexity of medical information. They may ask the doctor directly, "What do you recommend?" This question reflects the trust patients place in the physician's judgment.

The doctor's answer becomes the direction that shapes the next steps.

This decision-making role does not mean that doctors act alone.

Modern medicine encourages collaboration between healthcare professionals. Doctors frequently consult colleagues, review clinical guidelines, and discuss complex cases with specialists. Such collaboration strengthens the quality of decisions by incorporating diverse expertise.

However, even within collaborative environments, the doctor often remains the person responsible for guiding the final course of action.

This role places significant pressure on physicians.

Every decision carries consequences. Choosing one treatment may improve the patient's condition, while another option may introduce risks or complications. Even when decisions are made carefully, outcomes can sometimes remain uncertain because human biology does not always behave predictably.

Doctors must therefore make decisions with incomplete information while knowing that their choices affect real lives.

This responsibility contributes to the stabilizing role described in this chapter. When patients and families encounter uncertainty, they look toward the doctor as the individual capable of interpreting the situation and providing direction.

The physician's ability to remain calm and analytical during such moments helps create stability within the healthcare system.

Even when the outcome cannot be guaranteed, the presence of a professional who can evaluate possibilities and recommend a path forward reduces confusion and fear.

In this sense, the doctor functions as a central node in the decision-making process—a point where knowledge, responsibility, and trust converge to guide the uncertain journey from illness toward recovery.

7.3 — Stabilizing Patient Emotions

Illness rarely affects only the body. It also disrupts the emotional balance of the patient and often the entire family surrounding them. When symptoms appear or a diagnosis is suspected, fear, confusion, and anxiety quickly follow. People begin to imagine possibilities that they do not fully understand, and uncertainty can grow rapidly.

In such moments, the doctor's role extends beyond diagnosing disease.

The physician often becomes a stabilizing presence for the patient's emotional state. While the patient may feel overwhelmed by uncertainty, the doctor approaches the situation with experience and professional composure. This difference in perspective can create a powerful calming effect.

Patients watch the doctor carefully during consultations.

The tone of voice, the pace of explanation, and the confidence with which the physician speaks all influence how patients interpret their situation. A calm and structured conversation can reduce anxiety even before treatment begins.

For example, a patient who arrives fearing a serious illness may feel immediate relief when the doctor explains that the condition appears manageable. Even when the diagnosis is significant, the doctor's ability to explain the situation clearly can transform panic into understanding.

Clarity often replaces uncertainty.

Families also look to doctors for emotional direction. When relatives gather around a patient, their reactions can amplify each other's fears. One family member may imagine the worst outcome, while another may struggle to interpret medical information.

The doctor's explanation often becomes the point that brings these emotions back into balance.

A physician who communicates patiently can guide families from confusion toward cooperation. By outlining the condition, the available treatments, and the expected course of recovery, the doctor provides a framework that helps everyone involved understand what is happening.

This process restores a sense of control.

The stabilizing influence of doctors does not come only from words. It also comes from the attitude doctors display during difficult moments. Patients facing surgery, serious illness, or uncertain diagnoses often observe the doctor's demeanor closely.

If the physician remains calm and focused, patients often feel reassured that the situation is being handled competently.

In many cases, the doctor's confidence becomes a therapeutic force in itself.

When patients trust the doctor's judgment, they are more likely to follow treatment plans and cooperate with medical procedures. This cooperation improves the effectiveness of treatment and strengthens the partnership between doctor and patient.

Emotional stability therefore becomes an important element of healing.

However, maintaining this stabilizing presence requires effort from the doctor. Physicians must often manage their own emotional responses while supporting the patient's. They may encounter suffering, fear, and grief repeatedly throughout their work.

Despite these experiences, they are expected to remain composed.

This emotional discipline is part of the professional identity of doctors. Training teaches physicians to focus on solutions rather than panic, to approach illness analytically even when situations are emotionally charged.

In doing so, doctors create a space where patients can regain confidence.

When a patient enters the consultation room feeling anxious and leaves with a clearer understanding of their condition, something important has occurred. The doctor has not only provided medical guidance but also helped restore emotional balance.

This stabilizing role may not always be visible in medical records or clinical reports.

Yet it remains one of the most powerful contributions doctors make within the healthcare system. By helping patients and families move from fear toward understanding, physicians help transform illness from a moment of chaos into a situation that can be managed with knowledge, cooperation, and hope.

7.4 — The Bridge Between Knowledge and Humanity

Modern medicine is built upon an immense body of scientific knowledge. Research laboratories, universities, and medical institutions continuously expand our understanding of the human body and the diseases that affect it. Advances in genetics, pharmacology, imaging technologies, and surgical techniques have made it possible to diagnose and treat conditions that once seemed impossible to manage.

Yet this scientific knowledge is highly specialized.

Medical research is written in technical language, filled with complex terminology and detailed data that only trained professionals can fully interpret. For patients and families, this knowledge can feel distant and difficult to understand. When someone becomes ill, they rarely approach the situation with the scientific framework that doctors possess.

This is where the doctor's role becomes essential.

The physician acts as a bridge between the world of medical science and the everyday reality of human life. Doctors study complex biological processes for years so that they can interpret what is happening inside the body and translate that understanding into meaningful guidance for patients.

Without this translation, scientific knowledge would remain inaccessible to most people.

When a patient receives a diagnosis, the doctor does more than simply name the disease. The physician explains what the condition means, how it affects the body, and what steps can be taken to manage or treat it. This explanation transforms abstract scientific knowledge into practical understanding.

The doctor converts medical complexity into human language.

For example, a laboratory report may contain numerous technical measurements—levels of certain chemicals in the blood, patterns in imaging scans, or microscopic findings from tissue samples. To a patient, these details may appear confusing or even frightening.

The doctor interprets these results and places them into context.

A physician may explain that a particular test result indicates inflammation, that a scan shows a condition that can be treated, or that certain values fall within normal ranges. By translating technical information into clear explanations, the doctor helps the patient understand what is happening inside their body.

This translation reduces uncertainty.

It allows patients to see their illness not as an incomprehensible threat but as a condition that can be understood and addressed. Knowledge becomes accessible, and the patient gains the ability to participate actively in decisions about treatment.

The doctor's role as a bridge extends beyond explaining test results.

Doctors also connect medical science with the personal circumstances of patients. A treatment plan must consider not only what is scientifically effective but also what is practical within the patient's life. The physician must interpret medical knowledge in ways that align with the patient's responsibilities, financial resources, and emotional readiness.

This balancing act requires both scientific expertise and human awareness.

For example, a treatment may be medically ideal but difficult for the patient to follow because of work responsibilities or family obligations. The doctor must recognize these realities and help find solutions that maintain the effectiveness of treatment while respecting the patient's situation.

In doing so, the physician becomes more than a technical expert.

The doctor becomes a guide who helps patients navigate the complex intersection of science and daily life. Medical knowledge moves from textbooks and research papers into real-world decisions that shape how people recover and continue living.

This bridging role also strengthens trust.

Patients may not fully understand the scientific mechanisms behind their treatment, but they rely on the doctor to interpret that knowledge responsibly. The physician's ability to explain and guide becomes a vital link connecting the abstract world of medical research with the lived experience of illness.

Within the participatory field of healthcare, this role places doctors at a unique point of connection.

They stand between science and humanity, translating knowledge into care and transforming complex medical understanding into actions that support healing.

7.5 — The Responsibility of Trust

Trust is one of the most powerful forces in the relationship between doctors and society. When a patient enters a consultation room, they do so with an expectation that the physician will act with competence, honesty, and care. This trust allows patients to share deeply personal information about their bodies and their lives, often in moments of vulnerability.

Such openness is not easily given.

Patients describe symptoms that may be embarrassing or frightening. They allow doctors to examine them physically and to make decisions about treatments that may affect their future health. In many cases, patients follow medical advice even when they do not fully understand the scientific reasoning behind it.

This willingness to rely on the doctor's judgment is built upon trust.

For doctors, this trust is both an honor and a responsibility. The authority granted to physicians by society is not simply a privilege—it is a commitment to act in the best interests of those who seek help.

Medical ethics reflect this responsibility clearly.

From the earliest days of professional training, doctors are reminded that their knowledge must be used with integrity. They are expected to place patient welfare above personal gain, to provide accurate information, and to treat individuals with fairness and respect regardless of background or social status.

These ethical expectations exist because the consequences of broken trust can be profound.

When patients trust their doctors, they are more likely to follow treatment plans, report symptoms honestly, and cooperate during recovery. This cooperation strengthens the effectiveness of medical care and allows doctors to perform their role effectively.

But when trust is weakened, the entire healthcare system becomes unstable.

Patients who doubt the intentions of doctors may hesitate to follow medical advice. They may delay treatment, question recommendations, or seek multiple opinions without confidence in any of them. This uncertainty can slow the healing process and create tension between doctors and patients.

For doctors, maintaining trust requires constant awareness.

Clinical competence alone is not enough. The way physicians communicate, the transparency of their decisions, and the respect they show to patients all contribute to how trust is perceived. A doctor who explains a diagnosis clearly and listens to concerns patiently reinforces confidence in the medical relationship.

Even small actions can influence this perception.

A moment of attentiveness during a consultation, a careful explanation of treatment options, or a respectful response to a patient's question can strengthen trust significantly. These gestures remind patients that their well-being is genuinely valued.

At the same time, doctors must navigate challenges that can threaten this trust.

Modern healthcare systems involve financial pressures, administrative demands, and institutional constraints. Patients may sometimes feel that these forces influence medical decisions. When such perceptions arise, doctors must work carefully to demonstrate that patient welfare remains their primary concern.

The responsibility of trust therefore extends beyond individual consultations.

Doctors must uphold professional integrity not only in their interactions with patients but also in how they engage with the broader healthcare system. Ethical decision-making, transparency, and accountability help ensure that society continues to view the medical profession as reliable and honorable.

When trust is preserved, the doctor's role as a stabilizing node within healthcare becomes stronger.

Patients feel secure placing their health in the physician's hands. Families accept medical guidance with confidence. The healthcare system functions with cooperation rather than suspicion.

In this way, the responsibility of trust becomes one of the most important foundations upon which the entire practice of medicine rests.

7.6 — When the Stabilizing Node Weakens

The stabilizing role of doctors depends largely on trust. When patients believe that physicians are knowledgeable, ethical, and committed to their well-being, the doctor's presence brings clarity and reassurance into moments of uncertainty. The healthcare system functions smoothly because patients, families, and institutions align around the guidance that doctors provide.

But trust, once weakened, can disturb this balance.

In recent years, many healthcare systems have begun experiencing subtle shifts in the relationship between doctors and patients. Suspicion sometimes replaces confidence. Patients may approach consultations with doubts about motives, and doctors may feel that their decisions are constantly questioned.

This change does not occur suddenly.

Often it begins with small misunderstandings. A patient may leave the consultation feeling that the doctor did not listen carefully enough. A doctor may feel frustrated when a patient ignores important medical advice. These experiences accumulate over time, gradually influencing how both sides perceive each other.

Systemic pressures also contribute to this weakening of trust.

Modern healthcare environments are frequently busy and resource-constrained. Doctors may need to see many patients in a short period of time, leaving limited space for detailed conversations. Patients, however, often expect personal attention and clear explanations during consultations.

When these expectations are not met, dissatisfaction can arise.

Patients may interpret short consultations as indifference, while doctors may see them as necessary adaptations to institutional demands. This difference in perception can slowly erode the emotional stability that doctors traditionally provide within the healthcare system.

Public narratives sometimes amplify these tensions.

Stories about medical errors, negligence, or conflicts between doctors and patients can spread rapidly through media and social networks. While such cases represent only a small portion of medical practice, they can influence public perception strongly.

People may begin to view doctors with caution rather than confidence.

Doctors themselves are aware of this shift. The growing possibility of complaints, legal challenges, or public criticism can make physicians more cautious in their interactions. Some may adopt defensive approaches to treatment decisions, focusing more on protecting themselves from accusations than on maintaining open dialogue with patients.

This defensive posture can unintentionally increase emotional distance.

Patients who sense this distance may interpret it as lack of empathy, while doctors may feel that their professionalism is not fully recognized. The stabilizing node begins to weaken because the relationship between participants becomes strained.

The consequences of weakened trust extend beyond individual consultations.

Families may hesitate to accept medical advice without seeking multiple opinions. Patients may rely more heavily on informal information sources rather than professional guidance. Doctors may feel discouraged or emotionally exhausted when their efforts are met with suspicion.

In such conditions, the healthcare system loses some of the stability that doctors traditionally provide.

Understanding this process is important because it reveals that the weakening of trust is rarely caused by one side alone. It emerges from a combination of pressures—systemic limitations, communication gaps, rising expectations, and the emotional vulnerability that illness creates.

Each of these factors influences how doctors and patients perceive one another.

Recognizing these dynamics allows healthcare systems to address the problem more constructively. Strengthening communication, improving institutional support, and fostering mutual understanding between doctors and patients can help restore the stabilizing role that physicians have long played within society.

Because when trust between doctors and the public begins to fade, the entire field of healthcare becomes less stable.

7.7 — Rebuilding the Stabilizing Role

When the stabilizing role of doctors weakens, the entire healthcare system begins to feel the effects. Trust becomes fragile, communication becomes cautious, and the relationship between doctors and patients grows strained. Rebuilding this stability requires more than simply reminding doctors of their responsibilities or asking patients to be more trusting.

It requires a collective effort from all participants in the healthcare field.

The first step toward restoring stability lies in communication.

Doctors hold immense knowledge about the human body and disease, but patients often encounter medicine during moments of fear and uncertainty. When medical explanations remain technical or brief, patients may feel confused about their condition and uncertain about the path forward.

Clear and patient communication helps bridge this gap.

When doctors explain diagnoses, treatment options, and possible outcomes in language that patients can understand, confidence begins to grow. Patients who feel informed are more likely to cooperate with treatment and trust the decisions being made.

Communication does not require lengthy conversations. Sometimes a brief explanation delivered with clarity and attentiveness can transform how a patient perceives the entire consultation.

Professional humility also plays an important role.

Doctors are trained to guide medical decisions, but acknowledging uncertainty when it exists can strengthen rather than weaken trust. Patients often appreciate honesty about the limits of medical knowledge. When physicians openly explain what is known, what remains uncertain, and what steps will follow, patients feel included in the process rather than excluded from it.

This transparency restores balance in the relationship.

Institutions must also support doctors in maintaining their stabilizing role. Hospitals and healthcare systems that overwhelm physicians with excessive workloads or administrative pressures unintentionally weaken the doctor–patient relationship.

When doctors are given reasonable time to engage with patients and adequate resources to perform their duties, they are better able to fulfill the stabilizing role society expects from them.

Patients and families also contribute to rebuilding stability.

Trust cannot exist in only one direction. Patients who approach doctors with openness and honesty help create an environment where accurate diagnosis and treatment become possible. Recognizing that doctors operate within complex systems encourages patience and understanding when difficulties arise.

Healthcare works best when both sides see each other as partners rather than adversaries.

Society itself plays a role in shaping this partnership.

Public narratives about medicine influence how people approach healthcare interactions. Balanced discussions about both the achievements and the limitations of medical practice help create realistic expectations. When society recognizes that medicine involves both remarkable progress and unavoidable uncertainty, the doctor's role becomes easier to sustain.

Ultimately, rebuilding the stabilizing role of doctors is not about returning to a past where physicians were viewed as unquestioned authorities.

Instead, it involves creating a mature partnership between doctors, patients, institutions, and society. In this partnership, knowledge is respected, responsibility is shared, and communication remains open.

Within such a system, the doctor once again becomes a stabilizing node—not through authority alone, but through trust, clarity, and collaboration.

This renewed stability allows the healthcare system to function with greater harmony, ensuring that when illness disrupts human life, there remains a reliable center capable of guiding people back toward health.

The Weight of the White Coat

The white coat is often seen as a simple symbol of the medical profession. It represents education, scientific knowledge, and the authority that comes with years of training. Patients recognize it instantly, and its presence in a hospital or clinic often signals that help is available.

But the white coat carries a deeper meaning.

When a doctor puts on this coat, they do not merely step into a profession. They step into a position of responsibility that touches some of the most vulnerable moments of human life. People seek medical help when they are in pain, when they are uncertain about their future, or when someone they love is suffering.

In those moments, the doctor becomes more than a specialist.

The physician becomes the person who must bring clarity into confusion, calm into fear, and direction into uncertainty. A diagnosis organizes scattered symptoms into understanding. A treatment plan transforms anxiety into purposeful action.

Even when medicine cannot offer immediate solutions, the doctor's presence itself can restore a sense of stability.

This stabilizing role is not always visible.

Medical textbooks describe diseases, treatments, and procedures, but they rarely capture the emotional weight that doctors carry. Physicians must often make difficult decisions under pressure, communicate serious diagnoses with compassion, and continue working even after witnessing suffering that would overwhelm many others.

The white coat therefore represents both knowledge and endurance.

It symbolizes the expectation that doctors will remain steady when others feel uncertain. Patients and families often look to physicians not only for medical answers but also for reassurance that the situation can be managed.

In this sense, the white coat becomes a quiet anchor within the healthcare system.

Yet this responsibility should not be misunderstood as perfection. Doctors are human beings working within complex institutions and under demanding conditions. They face the same emotional and practical pressures that exist in other professions, often amplified by the life-and-death consequences of their work.

Recognizing this humanity is important.

When society views doctors only as technical experts, it overlooks the human dimension of the profession. The stabilizing role of physicians does not arise from authority alone; it arises from a combination of knowledge, responsibility, discipline, and empathy.

These qualities allow doctors to stand at the center of the healthcare system with credibility.

The white coat therefore represents a unique position in society. It marks the individual who must bridge science and humanity, who must guide patients through uncertainty, and who must uphold the trust that allows medicine to function effectively.

This weight cannot be carried by knowledge alone.

It is sustained by the commitment to remain steady when others are afraid, to act responsibly when decisions are difficult, and to remember that every case represents a human life seeking relief from suffering.

When doctors embrace this responsibility, the white coat becomes more than a professional uniform.

It becomes a symbol of stability within a system where science, trust, and human vulnerability meet—reminding both doctors and society that medicine, at its core, is not only about treating disease but about sustaining the fragile balance that allows healing to occur.

Chapter 8 — The Collapse of Trust

When Trust Begins to Crack

For a long time, the relationship between doctors and patients rested on a quiet foundation of trust. When illness appeared, people would seek the advice of a physician with the belief that the doctor possessed both the knowledge and the intention to help them recover. The consultation room was a place where fear met reassurance and uncertainty met guidance.

Patients rarely questioned the motives of the doctor.

They might not fully understand the diagnosis or the treatment plan, but they trusted that the physician's judgment was guided by experience and responsibility. Families accepted medical advice with confidence, and the authority of doctors was generally respected within society.

This trust allowed the healthcare system to function smoothly.

Doctors could focus on diagnosis and treatment without constant suspicion. Patients could concentrate on recovery rather than worrying about the intentions behind medical recommendations. Even when outcomes were uncertain, the presence of trust helped maintain stability in the relationship.

But over time, this foundation has begun to show signs of strain.

Today, interactions between doctors and patients sometimes begin with hesitation rather than confidence. Patients may arrive with doubts shaped by previous experiences, public narratives, or information gathered from the internet. Doctors may feel that their professional judgment is being questioned more frequently than before.

This shift does not occur because trust has suddenly disappeared.

Instead, it often weakens gradually through a series of small experiences. A rushed consultation, a misunderstanding about treatment costs, or a story about medical negligence shared through media can influence how patients approach future interactions with healthcare professionals.

These experiences accumulate quietly.

Patients may begin to wonder whether every recommended test is truly necessary. Doctors may feel frustrated when their clinical judgment is doubted before it is even explained. The atmosphere of cooperation that once defined the doctor–patient relationship becomes more cautious and guarded.

Both sides sense the change.

Patients sometimes feel that doctors are less attentive or more focused on institutional procedures. Doctors sometimes feel that patients approach them with suspicion rather than openness. The consultation room, which once felt like a space of trust, can begin to feel like a place where both sides must defend their positions.

This transformation reflects deeper changes within society.

Healthcare systems have become larger and more complex. Medical treatments are more advanced but also more expensive. Information about medicine is now widely available through digital platforms, allowing patients to access knowledge that was once limited to professionals.

While these developments have many benefits, they also alter how people perceive medical authority.

Trust, therefore, does not collapse in a single moment. It gradually erodes when expectations, communication, and experiences fail to align. Each misunderstanding adds a small crack to the foundation of the doctor–patient relationship.

Over time, these cracks become visible.

Understanding how this erosion occurs is essential for anyone who wishes to preserve the integrity of healthcare. Because medicine relies not only on scientific knowledge but also on the invisible bond of trust that allows patients and doctors to work together toward the same goal.

When that bond begins to weaken, the entire system feels the strain.

8.1 — The Changing Expectations of Patients

The expectations that patients bring into a medical consultation today are very different from those of earlier generations. In the past, people often approached doctors with a sense of unquestioned trust. Medical knowledge was largely inaccessible to the general public, and the doctor's advice was usually accepted without extensive discussion.

Patients assumed that the physician knew what was best.

This dynamic has gradually changed as society itself has changed. Access to information has expanded dramatically through the internet, digital health platforms, and social media. Today, patients frequently arrive at the clinic after reading about symptoms, possible diagnoses, and treatment options online.

Many patients conduct their own preliminary research before meeting the doctor.

This development has positive aspects. Patients who are informed about their health may ask thoughtful questions, understand treatment plans more clearly, and participate more actively in managing their conditions. Greater awareness about medical conditions can help individuals seek treatment earlier and follow preventive health practices.

However, increased access to information also changes how patients interpret medical authority.

When patients encounter multiple sources of medical information, they may begin comparing these sources with the advice given by the doctor. Differences between what they have read and what the physician recommends can create confusion or doubt.

Patients may wonder whether their online information is incomplete or whether the doctor's recommendation might be influenced by other factors.

In some cases, this comparison leads to constructive conversations. Patients ask questions, and doctors provide explanations that deepen understanding. But in other situations, the presence of conflicting information can weaken confidence in the doctor's judgment.

The consultation room becomes a space of negotiation rather than guidance.

Another factor shaping modern patient expectations is the advancement of medical technology. Over the past few decades, medicine has achieved remarkable successes—complex surgeries, life-saving drugs, and sophisticated diagnostic tools. These achievements have improved survival rates and extended life expectancy.

As a result, patients often expect modern medicine to solve most health problems quickly and effectively.

When treatment outcomes fall short of these expectations, disappointment can arise. Patients may feel that something has gone wrong or that better care should have been possible. The natural uncertainty of biology can sometimes clash with the expectation of technological precision.

Medicine, however, still operates within limits.

Some diseases remain difficult to treat. Recovery times may vary depending on individual conditions. Even highly advanced technologies cannot eliminate every risk associated with illness or treatment.

Understanding these limits is not always easy for patients who hope for clear and immediate solutions.

Social and economic factors also influence patient expectations. Healthcare today is often expensive, and patients who invest significant financial resources into treatment may naturally expect correspondingly strong results.

The perception of healthcare as a paid service can subtly transform the doctor–patient relationship.

Patients may begin to view medical consultations in transactional terms. If treatment outcomes are uncertain or communication feels insufficient, frustration may arise more quickly than in earlier generations where the relationship was framed primarily as professional guidance rather than service delivery.

These evolving expectations do not necessarily mean that patients trust doctors less by default.

Rather, patients now approach healthcare with greater awareness, more questions, and higher expectations about outcomes and communication. This shift requires doctors to engage with patients differently, providing clearer explanations and acknowledging the concerns that arise from modern access to information.

The doctor–patient relationship is therefore entering a new phase.

Trust is no longer based solely on authority. It increasingly depends on dialogue, transparency, and mutual understanding. Doctors must recognize that patients today seek participation in decisions about their health, while patients must recognize the complexity and uncertainty that physicians manage in clinical practice.

Navigating these changing expectations is essential for preserving trust within the healthcare system.

Because when expectations and communication align, informed patients and knowledgeable doctors can work together more effectively toward the shared goal of restoring health.

8.2 — The Pressure on Doctors in Modern Healthcare

While patients today approach healthcare with evolving expectations, doctors themselves are practicing in environments that have become increasingly complex. Modern healthcare systems involve advanced technologies, administrative procedures, regulatory requirements, and large patient populations.

These factors place significant pressure on physicians.

In many hospitals and clinics, doctors must attend to a high number of patients within limited time. Outpatient departments often receive dozens or even hundreds of patients in a single day. Each consultation requires listening to symptoms, reviewing medical history, examining the patient, interpreting test results, and deciding on a treatment plan.

Yet the available time for each interaction is often very short.

This situation creates a difficult balance. Patients expect detailed explanations and personal attention, but doctors must manage their responsibilities efficiently to ensure that every patient receives care. Even when physicians wish to spend more time discussing a case, institutional schedules and waiting patients may not allow it.

The result can be a consultation that feels rushed.

From the patient's perspective, a short consultation may appear as lack of interest or empathy. From the doctor's perspective, it may simply reflect the practical constraints of a busy healthcare environment. This difference in perception can quietly weaken the relationship between doctors and patients.

Administrative responsibilities add another layer of pressure.

Modern healthcare requires doctors to document patient histories, update electronic records, complete insurance forms, follow regulatory guidelines, and coordinate with hospital management systems. These tasks are essential for maintaining organized and accountable healthcare services.

However, they also consume time and mental energy.

A physician may spend a considerable portion of the workday completing documentation and administrative processes rather than engaging directly with patients. While these activities support the functioning of healthcare institutions, they can reduce the time available for meaningful doctor–patient communication.

Doctors must also stay updated with rapidly evolving medical knowledge.

Medical science advances continuously through research and technological innovation. New treatments, diagnostic techniques, and clinical guidelines emerge regularly. Physicians must dedicate time to learning and updating their knowledge so that they can provide accurate and effective care.

This ongoing learning is essential but demanding.

In addition to clinical responsibilities and administrative tasks, doctors often work long hours. Emergency cases, night duties, and unexpected complications can extend working days far beyond regular schedules. Over time, such demands can lead to physical fatigue and mental exhaustion.

Despite these pressures, doctors are expected to maintain composure and precision in their decisions.

Patients may encounter physicians during moments of exhaustion without realizing the workload that preceded the consultation. A doctor who appears distracted or brief in communication may simply be managing the cumulative pressures of a demanding work environment.

These pressures do not excuse poor communication, but they help explain why misunderstandings sometimes occur.

Modern healthcare therefore places doctors at the intersection of multiple responsibilities. They must diagnose and treat patients, manage institutional procedures, remain updated with scientific developments, and maintain ethical standards in every decision.

At the same time, they must preserve trust and empathy in their interactions with patients.

This combination of expectations creates a challenging environment. Doctors must perform complex intellectual and emotional tasks while working within systems that are often stretched by growing healthcare demands.

Understanding these pressures is important when examining the collapse of trust between doctors and patients.

Because when institutional constraints limit communication and attention, patients may feel neglected even when doctors are working intensely to provide the best care possible within the available circumstances.

8.3 — The Rise of Suspicion

As expectations change and pressures increase within healthcare systems, a subtle but important shift has begun to appear in the relationship between patients and doctors. In many places, consultations no longer begin with automatic trust. Instead, a small layer of suspicion sometimes enters the interaction even before the conversation begins.

Patients today often approach healthcare with questions that go beyond their symptoms.

They may wonder whether every recommended test is truly necessary, whether a particular medicine is the best option, or whether the doctor's advice might be influenced by financial or institutional incentives. These doubts do not always arise from personal experience; they are often shaped by stories circulating in society.

Public discussions about healthcare frequently highlight cases where treatment costs were excessive or where unnecessary procedures were allegedly recommended.

Even when such cases represent a small minority of medical practice, they can influence how patients perceive the entire profession. Stories of negative experiences travel quickly through communities, social media, and news platforms. Each story adds another layer to the collective perception of healthcare.

Gradually, suspicion becomes part of the background environment.

Patients may arrive at the consultation already prepared to evaluate the doctor's recommendations carefully. They might compare the advice with information found online or discuss it with friends and relatives before accepting it fully. What was once a relationship built primarily on trust begins to resemble a process of verification.

From the patient's perspective, this behavior may feel like caution rather than distrust.

Healthcare decisions can involve significant financial costs and emotional consequences. Patients often feel responsible for protecting themselves and their families from mistakes or unnecessary treatments. Asking questions and seeking additional information may seem like a reasonable approach.

However, from the doctor's perspective, this shift can feel different.

Physicians may sense that their professional judgment is being questioned before it is fully explained. When patients approach consultations with skepticism, doctors may feel that the trust traditionally associated with their profession is gradually diminishing.

This atmosphere can subtly change the tone of interactions.

Doctors may become more careful in how they present recommendations, anticipating doubts that may arise. Patients may interpret this caution as uncertainty or hesitation. Both sides attempt to protect themselves, and the openness that once defined the doctor–patient relationship begins to weaken.

The rise of suspicion also affects how patients interpret medical advice.

For example, when a doctor recommends diagnostic tests, patients may wonder whether the tests are necessary for diagnosis or simply part of routine hospital procedures. When medicines are prescribed, some patients may question whether alternative options exist that were not mentioned.

These doubts can slow the process of decision-making.

Instead of moving directly toward treatment, patients may seek multiple opinions or delay decisions while evaluating information from various sources. While second opinions can sometimes improve understanding, excessive doubt can also prolong uncertainty and complicate treatment.

Suspicion therefore creates a difficult environment for both sides.

Patients may feel that they must protect themselves from potential mistakes or financial burdens. Doctors may feel that their professional integrity is being judged continuously. The consultation room becomes a space where both participants carry a degree of caution.

Understanding the rise of suspicion is important because it reveals that the erosion of trust is not always driven by direct conflict.

Often it emerges quietly from broader social narratives, economic concerns, and the growing availability of medical information. Each of these influences shapes how patients approach doctors and how doctors respond in return.

The challenge for modern healthcare lies in finding ways to transform suspicion back into constructive dialogue.

When patients feel comfortable asking questions and doctors feel respected while providing explanations, suspicion can gradually give way to understanding. Trust, once weakened, can begin to rebuild through transparency, communication, and shared responsibility in the process of care.

8.4 — Defensive Medicine

As mistrust slowly enters the doctor–patient relationship, it begins to influence how doctors practice medicine itself. One of the most significant consequences of this change is the rise of what is often called *defensive medicine.*

Defensive medicine occurs when doctors make medical decisions not only based on clinical judgment, but also with the intention of protecting themselves from possible complaints, accusations, or legal action.

In earlier times, physicians primarily focused on identifying the disease and selecting the most appropriate treatment. Today, many doctors must also consider another question alongside their clinical reasoning:

"How will this decision appear if it is questioned later?"

This additional layer of caution subtly reshapes medical practice.

Doctors may order more diagnostic tests than strictly necessary, not because the tests will change the treatment plan, but because having more documented evidence can help protect the physician if the case is later scrutinized. Additional tests create a record showing that the doctor explored every possible angle.

From the doctor's perspective, this documentation acts as a safeguard.

For patients, however, the situation may appear differently. When multiple tests are recommended, patients sometimes interpret them as unnecessary or financially motivated. The very action intended to protect the doctor can inadvertently strengthen patient suspicion.

A cycle begins to form.

Doctors recommend additional tests to protect themselves. Patients begin to suspect that tests are unnecessary. This suspicion further encourages doctors to practice defensively.

The relationship gradually moves away from pure clinical trust.

Defensive medicine also affects treatment decisions. In uncertain situations, doctors may choose options that are legally safer rather than medically simpler. For example, referring a patient to multiple specialists or recommending hospitalization for observation may reduce personal risk for the physician.

These choices often arise from caution rather than medical necessity.

Doctors operate in environments where a single negative outcome—sometimes unavoidable in medicine—can lead to complaints, investigations, or legal disputes. Even when a physician has acted responsibly, the stress of defending a medical decision can be significant.

To avoid such situations, doctors sometimes take extra precautions.

Over time, this defensive mindset can change the emotional atmosphere of medical practice. Instead of focusing entirely on patient care, doctors must constantly think about documentation, legal implications, and how each decision might be interpreted later.

This adds another layer of mental pressure to an already demanding profession.

Patients may also sense this shift.

A doctor who focuses heavily on documentation, forms, and test reports may appear distant or overly procedural. The human conversation that once characterized the doctor–patient relationship may feel replaced by a series of formal steps designed to protect both sides.

The irony is that defensive medicine often arises from a desire to maintain professional security, yet it can unintentionally weaken trust.

When consultations become heavily procedural, patients may feel that medicine is becoming mechanical rather than compassionate. Doctors, meanwhile, may feel that their professional judgment is constantly under scrutiny.

The stabilizing node begins to experience tension.

It is important to recognize that defensive medicine is rarely a result of individual intention alone. It emerges from the broader environment in which healthcare operates—legal frameworks, institutional policies, public expectations, and the increasing visibility of medical errors in public discussions.

Doctors respond to these pressures as professionals trying to protect themselves while continuing to provide care.

Understanding defensive medicine helps reveal an important truth about the collapse of trust: both sides are reacting to uncertainty.

Patients fear being misled or overcharged. Doctors fear being accused or misunderstood.

Both responses arise from the same underlying erosion of confidence.

Restoring trust therefore requires creating environments where doctors can practice medicine primarily according to clinical judgment, and where patients can feel confident that medical recommendations are guided by care rather than caution alone.

8.5 — Media Narratives and Public Perception

Public perception of the medical profession is shaped not only by personal experiences but also by the stories that circulate through society. In earlier generations, most people formed their understanding of doctors primarily through direct interactions within their communities. A physician who treated families for years became a familiar and trusted figure.

Today, however, media plays a powerful role in shaping how people view healthcare.

News reports, television programs, social media discussions, and online platforms continuously present stories related to hospitals, medical treatments, and healthcare systems. These narratives influence how people interpret their own experiences with doctors and how they approach future medical consultations.

Media attention often focuses on extraordinary events.

Stories about successful surgeries, groundbreaking treatments, or medical discoveries highlight the remarkable achievements of modern medicine. At the same time, reports about medical negligence, disputes between patients and hospitals, or controversial treatment decisions receive significant public attention.

Negative stories tend to travel particularly quickly.

When a case of alleged malpractice appears in the news or spreads through social media, it can reach thousands or even millions of people within a short period. These stories often evoke strong emotional reactions, especially when they involve suffering patients or grieving families.

For many viewers or readers, such stories become symbolic examples of larger problems within the healthcare system.

Even though most medical interactions occur without conflict, the dramatic nature of negative incidents makes them more visible and memorable. People may begin to associate these rare events with the entire profession, creating a perception that such incidents are more common than they actually are.

This phenomenon shapes expectations before patients even meet their doctors.

A patient who has recently heard several stories about medical negligence may approach a consultation with caution. They may interpret routine medical procedures or recommendations through the lens of those stories. Suspicion can arise not from personal experience but from narratives absorbed through media.

Doctors are aware of these narratives as well.

Physicians often recognize that public perception of their profession is influenced by widely shared stories. When media discussions portray healthcare primarily through the lens of conflict or controversy, doctors may feel that their work is being evaluated through isolated incidents rather than the broader reality of everyday medical practice.

This perception can affect how doctors engage with patients.

Physicians may become more cautious in communication or more attentive to documentation, anticipating that misunderstandings could escalate quickly in an environment shaped by intense public scrutiny.

Social media has intensified this dynamic further.

Unlike traditional media, where stories pass through editorial processes, social platforms allow individuals to share personal experiences instantly. A single post describing dissatisfaction with medical treatment can spread widely before the full context of the situation is understood.

Public opinion may form rapidly.

This immediacy sometimes creates an atmosphere where healthcare professionals feel that their decisions can be judged publicly without complete information. Patients, on the other hand, may feel empowered to share experiences that might otherwise remain private.

Both developments influence the evolving relationship between doctors and society.

The challenge lies in balancing transparency with fairness. Media discussions about healthcare are important because they highlight areas where improvement is needed. Accountability within medicine strengthens the profession when handled responsibly.

However, when narratives focus primarily on negative cases without context, they can distort public perception.

Patients may begin to see doctors through a lens of suspicion rather than trust. Doctors may feel that their dedication and hard work are overshadowed by isolated incidents.

The consultation room then carries the weight of these broader narratives.

Understanding the influence of media helps explain why mistrust sometimes grows even when most medical interactions remain respectful and constructive. Public perception does not always arise solely from direct experience; it is shaped by the stories society tells about medicine.

Rebuilding trust therefore requires not only better communication between doctors and patients but also a more balanced understanding of healthcare within public discussions.

8.6 — When Patients and Doctors Become Adversaries

At the heart of medicine lies a simple relationship: one person seeks help, and another offers knowledge and care. For generations, this relationship functioned largely as a partnership. Patients trusted doctors to guide them through illness, and doctors trusted patients to share symptoms honestly and follow medical advice.

But when trust weakens, the tone of this relationship can change.

Instead of approaching each other as partners in healing, patients and doctors may begin to see each other through a lens of caution or defensiveness. The consultation room, which should ideally be a space of cooperation, can slowly transform into a place where both sides feel the need to protect themselves.

This shift often begins subtly.

A patient may ask questions with a tone of suspicion rather than curiosity. A doctor may respond with guarded explanations, aware that every word could be interpreted critically. Both participants sense the tension but may not openly address it.

The interaction becomes more formal and less human.

Patients sometimes feel that doctors are distant or impatient. Doctors may feel that patients arrive with predetermined assumptions or doubts about their intentions. Each side begins to interpret the other's behavior in ways that reinforce mistrust.

Small misunderstandings can escalate quickly in this environment.

For example, if a patient believes that a doctor recommended unnecessary tests, frustration may arise even before the doctor has an opportunity to explain the medical reasoning behind the recommendation. If the doctor senses this frustration, the response may become more procedural and less conversational.

Communication begins to deteriorate.

Family members can also influence this dynamic. When relatives accompany a patient, they may express strong opinions about treatment decisions or question the doctor's advice. These reactions often arise from concern for the patient's well-being, but they can sometimes intensify tension in the consultation.

Doctors may feel that their professional judgment is being challenged.

Patients and families, meanwhile, may feel that their concerns are not being taken seriously. Each side believes it is defending something important—patients defend their health and financial security, while doctors defend their professional integrity and medical judgment.

The relationship gradually shifts from collaboration to confrontation.

In extreme cases, these tensions can lead to open conflict. Arguments may occur in hospitals or clinics, complaints may be filed against physicians, and the situation may attract public attention through media or social platforms.

When such conflicts occur, they reinforce the perception that doctors and patients stand on opposite sides.

This adversarial mindset is deeply damaging to healthcare.

Medicine functions best when doctors and patients work together with shared goals. When suspicion replaces cooperation, the quality of communication declines, and important details about symptoms or treatment may be overlooked.

Healing becomes more difficult in an atmosphere of conflict.

Doctors may become emotionally distant to protect themselves from confrontation. Patients may withhold trust or delay decisions while seeking additional reassurance. The stabilizing role that physicians traditionally play within healthcare becomes weakened.

Understanding this shift is essential because it reveals that adversarial relationships rarely arise from a single moment of disagreement.

They grow gradually through repeated experiences of miscommunication, unmet expectations, and social narratives that shape how each side views the other. When these influences accumulate, the partnership between doctor and patient begins to fracture.

Restoring cooperation requires recognizing that both sides ultimately seek the same outcome.

Patients want relief from illness and protection of their well-being. Doctors want to apply their knowledge to help restore health. When these shared intentions are acknowledged, the adversarial dynamic can begin to dissolve.

The consultation room can once again become a place where trust, dialogue, and cooperation guide the process of healing.

8.7 — Understanding the Shared Responsibility

When trust between doctors and patients begins to weaken, it is tempting to search for a single cause. Some may blame doctors for becoming too commercial or detached, while others may blame patients for becoming overly suspicious or demanding. Yet the reality is far more complex.

The erosion of trust rarely originates from one side alone.

It emerges from a combination of pressures, expectations, and experiences that influence both doctors and patients simultaneously. Understanding this shared responsibility is essential if the healthcare system is to regain stability.

Doctors today operate within environments that are more demanding than ever before. Large patient volumes, administrative requirements, evolving medical knowledge, and legal scrutiny all shape how physicians practice medicine. These pressures can limit the time available for communication and increase the mental burden placed on doctors.

Patients, on the other hand, approach healthcare with their own challenges.

Illness often brings fear, financial concerns, and emotional stress. When someone's health or the well-being of a loved one is at stake, even small uncertainties can feel overwhelming. Patients naturally seek reassurance and clarity during these moments.

If communication fails to meet these needs, frustration can arise.

Both sides therefore react to vulnerability in different ways. Doctors may become more cautious or procedural as they manage institutional pressures. Patients may become more questioning or skeptical as they try to protect themselves from potential risks.

Neither reaction is entirely unreasonable.

However, when these reactions occur simultaneously, they can reinforce each other. A cautious doctor may appear distant to the patient. A questioning patient may appear distrustful to the doctor. Each side interprets the other's behavior as confirmation of their own concerns.

The cycle of mistrust gradually strengthens.

Economic realities also influence this dynamic. Healthcare today often involves significant financial costs for patients. Medical education and hospital infrastructure also require large investments, which shape how healthcare institutions operate.

These financial dimensions can influence how people perceive medical decisions.

Patients may wonder whether certain tests or treatments are recommended purely for clinical reasons or influenced by institutional systems. Doctors, meanwhile, may feel that their professional judgment is being interpreted through the lens of financial suspicion.

This tension adds another layer to the collapse of trust.

Social narratives and media discussions further amplify these concerns. Public conversations about healthcare often highlight negative experiences, which can shape expectations before patients even meet their doctors.

Doctors and patients therefore enter consultations carrying perceptions influenced by broader societal conversations.

Recognizing shared responsibility helps move the discussion away from blame.

Doctors can reflect on how communication, empathy, and transparency influence patient trust. Patients can recognize the complexity of medical practice and the pressures doctors face while making difficult decisions.

When both sides acknowledge these realities, the relationship becomes more balanced.

Instead of viewing each other as opponents, doctors and patients can begin to see themselves as participants in the same process. Each side brings different knowledge and experiences to the consultation, and both contribute to the outcome of care.

Trust grows when responsibility is shared.

The doctor provides expertise and guidance. The patient provides honest information about symptoms and circumstances. Families offer support, and institutions create the environment in which care is delivered.

Together, these elements form the field within which healing becomes possible.

Understanding this shared responsibility is the first step toward rebuilding the trust that modern healthcare increasingly depends upon.

Trust as the Invisible Medicine

Medicine is often associated with powerful technologies, complex procedures, and advanced scientific knowledge. Hospitals contain sophisticated equipment capable of diagnosing diseases deep within the body. Laboratories analyze biological samples with remarkable precision. Pharmaceutical research continues to develop medicines that extend and improve human life.

Yet beneath all these visible elements lies something less tangible but equally essential.

Trust.

Trust rarely appears in medical reports or scientific studies, yet it quietly supports every successful interaction between doctors and patients. It allows patients to share symptoms honestly, to follow treatment recommendations, and to accept medical decisions even when outcomes remain uncertain.

Without trust, medicine becomes far more difficult.

A patient who doubts the doctor's intentions may hesitate to follow treatment advice. A doctor who feels constantly questioned may become cautious or distant in communication. Even the most advanced medical technology cannot compensate for a relationship weakened by suspicion.

Healing depends not only on science but also on cooperation.

When trust exists, the consultation room becomes a place where two participants work toward the same goal. The patient brings personal experience of illness, and the doctor brings professional knowledge. Together they create a shared understanding of the problem and a plan for recovery.

Trust allows this partnership to function smoothly.

However, trust is fragile. It grows slowly through repeated experiences of honesty, care, and professionalism. But it can weaken quickly when communication fails or expectations remain unmet.

The collapse of trust described in this chapter therefore deserves careful attention.

It does not represent a simple conflict between doctors and patients. Rather, it reflects the pressures and misunderstandings that arise when modern healthcare systems become complex and communication between participants begins to falter.

Recognizing this fragility offers an opportunity.

Doctors who communicate clearly and treat patients with respect strengthen the foundation of trust. Patients who approach consultations with openness and honesty contribute equally to this foundation. Institutions that support transparency and fairness help maintain the environment in which trust can thrive.

Each participant has a role in preserving it.

When trust is present, medicine becomes more effective. Patients cooperate more readily with treatment. Doctors can focus on clinical judgment rather than defensive caution. The healthcare system functions with greater stability.

Trust therefore acts like an invisible medicine within the healing process.

It does not cure disease directly, but it creates the conditions in which treatment can succeed. It transforms the consultation room from a place of uncertainty into a space where knowledge, responsibility, and hope can work together.

In the end, the strength of medicine does not depend only on scientific progress.

It depends equally on the fragile yet powerful bond of trust that connects doctors and patients in their shared effort to restore health.

Reflective Interlude

When the Field Becomes a System

Until this point, we have looked at medicine primarily through the human relationship between doctors and patients. We examined how doctors are shaped by training, how patients arrive with fear and expectation, and how trust acts as the invisible force holding the entire interaction together.

But the consultation room does not exist in isolation.

Every doctor–patient interaction occurs within a larger structure. Hospitals are institutions. Healthcare is regulated by governments. Insurance systems influence what treatments are affordable. Pharmaceutical companies develop medicines that become part of clinical practice.

Medicine therefore functions not only as a human relationship but also as a system.

And systems have their own dynamics.

Systems bring organization and scale. They allow hospitals to treat thousands of patients, coordinate complex procedures, and distribute medical knowledge across societies. Without systems, modern healthcare would not be possible.

Yet systems also introduce power.

When medicine becomes embedded in large institutional structures, decisions are no longer shaped solely by the doctor's clinical judgment or the patient's needs. Policies, budgets, regulations, corporate interests, and political priorities begin to influence how healthcare is delivered.

Gradually, the field of medicine becomes layered.

At the center lies the human relationship between doctor and patient. Surrounding that relationship are institutional systems—hospitals, insurance companies, pharmaceutical industries, regulatory bodies, and governments.

Each layer exerts influence.

Sometimes this influence strengthens healthcare. Organized systems can expand access to treatment, standardize medical practices, and support research that benefits millions of people.

But systems can also distort the original purpose of medicine.

Financial incentives may influence how hospitals operate. Institutional targets may shape how doctors allocate time to patients. Pharmaceutical marketing may affect how treatments are promoted. Regulatory pressures may alter how decisions are documented and defended.

None of these forces are inherently malicious.

They arise naturally as societies attempt to organize complex healthcare systems. Yet over time, they can gradually shift the center of medicine away from the human relationship that once defined it.

Doctors begin to feel constrained by systems. Patients begin to feel processed by institutions. Trust becomes entangled in bureaucracy.

The doctor who once stood as a stabilizing node within the healthcare field may now appear as only one participant within a much larger machine.

This transformation is subtle but profound.

When systems grow powerful enough, the human connection between doctor and patient risks becoming secondary to the mechanisms that surround it. Efficiency, regulation, and institutional priorities can quietly overshadow the simple act of healing.

Understanding this transition is essential.

Because the collapse of trust we explored earlier is not only a matter of human misunderstanding. It is also a reflection of how healthcare systems have evolved and how power flows through those systems.

To understand medicine today, we must therefore look beyond the consultation room.

We must examine how systems shape decisions, how power influences priorities, and how the original purpose of medicine can sometimes become distorted within large institutional frameworks.

This brings us to the next stage of our exploration.

In next part we will examine how the structures surrounding healthcare influence doctors, patients, and the fragile trust that binds them together.

PART III — SYSTEM, POWER, AND DISTORTION

When systems grow in strength, they must be guided by awareness—or they begin to distort what they were meant to serve.

Chapter 9 — When Medicine Becomes a Market

From Healing to Industry

For centuries, medicine was largely understood as a profession centered on healing. Doctors worked in small clinics, community hospitals, or private practices where their primary responsibility was to diagnose illness and help restore health. The relationship between doctor and patient stood at the center of medical practice.

Economic considerations certainly existed, but they remained secondary to the purpose of care.

Patients paid for consultations, medicines, or procedures, yet the scale of healthcare systems was relatively limited. Medical technologies were simpler, hospital infrastructures were modest, and the costs associated with treatment were comparatively manageable.

The physician's role was defined primarily by knowledge and service.

Over time, however, medicine began to evolve alongside the broader transformation of modern society. Scientific discoveries expanded the possibilities of treatment. Advanced technologies allowed doctors to see inside the human body, perform complex surgeries, and develop powerful medicines capable of addressing diseases that once seemed untreatable.

These achievements dramatically improved human health.

But they also changed the structure of healthcare itself.

Modern hospitals now contain sophisticated imaging machines, intensive care units, robotic surgical systems, and specialized laboratories. Maintaining such infrastructure requires significant financial investment. The development of new medicines and medical devices involves years of research, testing, and regulatory approval.

Healthcare gradually became one of the most resource-intensive sectors of modern economies.

As systems expanded, institutions began organizing healthcare on a much larger scale. Hospitals grew into complex organizations employing hundreds or thousands of professionals. Administrative departments developed to manage finances, insurance systems, legal compliance, and operational logistics.

Medicine slowly moved from small community-based practice toward large institutional structures.

With this transformation came a new dimension: economics.

Healthcare systems needed sustainable financial models to support their infrastructure, technology, and workforce. Governments, private investors, insurance companies, and healthcare corporations all became participants in shaping how medical services were delivered.

Medicine therefore began to operate within the logic of markets.

Hospitals required revenue to maintain operations. Pharmaceutical companies invested heavily in research and development. Diagnostic laboratories expanded services and technologies. Insurance systems developed to manage the costs associated with treatment.

These economic structures allowed healthcare to expand and innovate.

At the same time, they also changed how medicine was perceived.

Patients increasingly encountered healthcare through institutions that resembled organized service systems. Bills, insurance claims, hospital packages, and pricing structures became part of the treatment experience. Financial conversations sometimes accompanied medical discussions.

The environment surrounding medicine began to resemble other sectors of the economy.

For doctors, this shift created new complexities. Physicians who entered the profession with the intention of practicing healing found themselves working within systems shaped by financial planning, operational targets, and institutional policies.

For patients, the experience of healthcare sometimes began to feel like participation in a marketplace.

People who paid significant amounts for treatment naturally expected clear results and accountability. Medical services began to be evaluated not only through the lens of care but also through the expectations associated with financial transactions.

This transformation did not occur because medicine lost its purpose.

It emerged as a consequence of progress itself. Scientific innovation, technological advancement, and large-scale healthcare systems brought tremendous benefits to humanity. But they also introduced economic forces that gradually reshaped how medicine operates.

Understanding this shift is essential.

Because when medicine becomes embedded within market structures, the delicate balance between care and commerce must be carefully maintained. If that balance tilts too far toward economic priorities, the human relationship between doctor and patient can begin to feel secondary.

The chapters that follow explore how this transformation unfolded—and how the forces of economics, institutions, and incentives continue to influence the practice of medicine today.

9.1 — The Economics of Modern Healthcare

Modern healthcare is often discussed in moral or professional terms—service, compassion, responsibility, and ethics. These elements remain central to the identity of medicine. Yet beneath these ideals lies another reality that is impossible to ignore: healthcare is also an economic system.

Treating illness requires resources.

Every consultation, diagnostic test, surgical procedure, or hospital admission depends on infrastructure, equipment, trained professionals, and supporting services. Unlike earlier centuries when medicine relied largely on observation and simple remedies, modern healthcare operates through complex scientific and technological systems.

These systems come with substantial costs.

Consider the path that leads someone to become a doctor. Medical education itself requires years of training, access to laboratories, clinical exposure, and specialized faculty. Universities and teaching hospitals invest enormous resources in training future physicians.

For many students, medical education also involves significant personal financial commitment.

Once doctors enter professional practice, the economic dimension of healthcare becomes even more visible. Hospitals require large physical infrastructures—buildings equipped with operating theatres, emergency departments, intensive care units, laboratories, imaging centers, and specialized wards.

Each component requires constant maintenance.

Advanced medical technologies also contribute significantly to healthcare costs. Machines such as MRI scanners, CT scanners, robotic surgical systems, and high-end diagnostic equipment represent major investments. These technologies must be purchased, maintained, upgraded, and operated by trained personnel.

While they improve diagnostic accuracy and treatment outcomes, they also increase operational expenses.

Healthcare institutions must also support a wide workforce beyond doctors. Nurses, technicians, pharmacists, administrators, support staff, biomedical engineers, and many others contribute to the functioning of hospitals and clinics.

Their training, salaries, and professional development form an essential part of healthcare economics.

Even the medicines that patients receive are products of complex economic processes. Pharmaceutical research requires years of scientific investigation, clinical trials, regulatory approvals, and manufacturing infrastructure. The cost of developing a single new drug can involve substantial investment before it ever reaches patients.

These investments shape the pricing structures of medical treatments.

Public healthcare systems funded by governments must allocate budgets carefully to sustain these services for large populations. Private healthcare systems must generate revenue to maintain operations and attract investment for future expansion.

In both cases, healthcare becomes closely connected to economic planning.

Patients encounter this economic reality in many ways. Diagnostic tests, hospital admissions, medications, and surgical procedures often involve financial considerations. Insurance systems have developed in many countries to help distribute these costs, but the underlying economics of healthcare remain significant.

This financial dimension influences how healthcare institutions operate.

Hospitals must balance the goal of providing quality care with the need to remain financially sustainable. Governments must design policies that ensure access to healthcare while managing national budgets. Insurance providers must calculate risks and premiums to support coverage systems.

Doctors practice medicine within this complex economic environment.

Most physicians do not directly control these financial structures, yet their daily work occurs within them. Treatment decisions may interact with insurance approvals, hospital policies, or institutional guidelines designed to manage costs.

Understanding the economics of modern healthcare does not diminish the ethical purpose of medicine.

Rather, it reveals the scale of the system required to deliver modern medical care. The extraordinary capabilities of contemporary medicine—from advanced surgeries to lifesaving medications—exist because societies have invested immense resources into building healthcare systems.

However, this economic foundation also introduces new tensions.

When healthcare becomes deeply embedded within financial structures, the challenge arises of ensuring that economic sustainability does not overshadow the primary purpose of medicine: caring for human life.

Maintaining this balance remains one of the central challenges of modern healthcare systems.

9.2 — Hospitals as Institutions, Not Just Clinics

In earlier times, healthcare was often delivered through small clinics or community-based medical practices. A doctor might treat patients in a modest facility with a limited number of beds, basic diagnostic tools, and a small supporting staff. The structure was simple, and the relationship between doctor and patient remained the central focus.

Modern hospitals are very different.

Today's hospitals operate as large and complex institutions. They resemble organized ecosystems where hundreds of professionals, technologies, and administrative systems work together to deliver healthcare. A single hospital may contain specialized departments for cardiology, neurology, oncology, orthopedics, emergency care, intensive care, and many other fields.

Each department functions with its own teams, equipment, and procedures.

Managing such an environment requires structured administration. Hospital management must coordinate staffing schedules, maintain medical equipment, regulate supply chains, oversee financial planning, ensure legal compliance, and maintain quality standards across departments.

These responsibilities transform hospitals into organizational systems rather than simple treatment centers.

In many cases, hospitals now operate with structures similar to large corporations. They have executive leadership, financial planning departments, human resource management, marketing teams, and operational strategies designed to sustain long-term growth.

These institutional frameworks are necessary for managing large-scale healthcare delivery.

Running a modern hospital involves enormous operational costs. Buildings must be maintained, advanced technologies must be serviced, and medical supplies must remain available at all times. Staffing requirements extend across multiple shifts to ensure continuous care.

Emergency departments, intensive care units, and surgical theatres must remain ready around the clock.

To sustain these operations, hospitals must develop financial models that support their infrastructure. Some institutions are funded by governments and public health systems. Others operate as private organizations supported by patient payments, insurance reimbursements, or investment capital.

In both cases, financial management becomes an essential component of hospital administration.

This institutional structure influences how healthcare is delivered.

Doctors working within hospitals often function as part of large teams rather than independent practitioners. Treatment decisions may involve collaboration with specialists, nursing teams, diagnostic units, and hospital administrators. Clinical protocols and institutional guidelines help standardize care across departments.

While these systems improve coordination, they also introduce new layers of complexity.

For patients, entering a hospital can sometimes feel like entering a large organization rather than visiting a personal clinic. Registration counters, billing departments, diagnostic scheduling, insurance processing, and multiple consultations may all become part of the treatment journey.

The experience of healthcare becomes institutional.

Doctors themselves must adapt to these environments. Physicians may spend time interacting not only with patients but also with hospital management systems, administrative requirements, and institutional procedures. Clinical decisions may intersect with hospital policies regarding documentation, resource allocation, or treatment protocols.

This does not necessarily mean that the purpose of medicine has changed.

Hospitals still exist to diagnose illness, treat disease, and restore health. The institutional structures surrounding them have evolved primarily to manage the scale and complexity of modern healthcare.

However, these structures also influence how medicine is practiced.

When healthcare operates within large institutions, the relationship between doctor and patient becomes one part of a broader system involving administrators, financial planners, regulatory authorities, and technological infrastructure.

Understanding this institutional dimension helps explain why modern medicine sometimes feels different from the traditional image of the doctor's clinic.

The physician remains a central figure in the healing process, but the environment in which that role is performed has expanded into a large and carefully organized institutional framework.

9.3 — The Pressure on Doctors Inside Institutions

When medicine becomes institutionalized, the role of the doctor also begins to change. Physicians who once worked as relatively independent practitioners now often operate within large organizational structures where many decisions are influenced by institutional systems.

Doctors still carry the responsibility of diagnosing illness and guiding treatment.

However, they must now perform these duties within environments shaped by hospital policies, administrative protocols, financial planning, and operational targets. These institutional frameworks influence how doctors organize their time, interact with patients, and manage clinical decisions.

One of the most visible pressures within institutional medicine is productivity.

Hospitals often measure performance through indicators such as patient volume, consultation numbers, surgical output, or departmental efficiency. These metrics help institutions evaluate how effectively healthcare services are being delivered.

For doctors, this can translate into expectations to see many patients within limited time.

A physician working in a busy hospital outpatient department may consult dozens of patients in a single day. Each consultation involves reviewing symptoms, examining the patient, considering diagnostic possibilities, and explaining treatment options.

Yet the time available for each interaction is often constrained by institutional schedules.

This environment can create tension between two important priorities: efficiency and attention.

Doctors may wish to spend more time listening to patients and explaining conditions carefully, but the institutional structure requires them to maintain a steady flow of consultations so that all waiting patients receive care. When time becomes limited, conversations may become shorter and more focused on clinical essentials.

Patients sometimes interpret this as lack of empathy.

In reality, many doctors are simply navigating the practical constraints of institutional healthcare systems. Physicians must balance their commitment to individual patients with their responsibility to ensure that the system continues to function for everyone.

Institutional medicine also introduces administrative expectations.

Doctors are required to maintain detailed documentation, complete electronic health records, follow hospital protocols, and coordinate with other departments. These processes are important for maintaining accountability and ensuring continuity of care.

However, they also occupy time that might otherwise be spent directly with patients.

Another form of pressure arises from hierarchical structures within institutions. Junior doctors often work under senior consultants, and decisions may pass through multiple levels of review. While this structure helps maintain clinical oversight, it can sometimes limit the autonomy of individual physicians.

Doctors must often align their decisions with departmental guidelines or institutional policies.

These pressures are not inherently negative.

Large healthcare institutions allow complex treatments to be performed safely and efficiently. Collaboration between specialists improves patient outcomes, and standardized protocols help maintain quality across departments.

Yet the institutional environment can sometimes create internal conflicts for doctors.

Physicians enter the profession with the intention of practicing healing and applying scientific knowledge for the benefit of patients. When institutional pressures shape how quickly consultations occur or how resources are allocated, doctors may feel that the human dimension of medicine becomes compressed by operational demands.

The challenge for modern healthcare systems is therefore delicate.

Institutions must remain efficient and financially sustainable while still allowing doctors the professional space necessary to practice thoughtful and compassionate medicine.

Understanding these pressures helps patients see that the doctor they meet in a hospital is not working alone.

The physician operates within a network of institutional forces that influence how healthcare is delivered. Recognizing this reality is important when examining the broader transformation of medicine into a structured and economically organized system.

9.4 — The Patient as a Consumer

As healthcare systems become increasingly structured around institutions, technologies, and financial models, the role of the patient also begins to change. In earlier forms of medical practice, patients were primarily viewed as individuals seeking guidance and care from a trusted physician.

The relationship was framed largely in professional and human terms.

Today, however, the economic structures surrounding healthcare sometimes reshape how patients perceive their role within the system. When medical treatment involves significant financial costs—consultation fees, diagnostic tests, hospital charges, and medication expenses—patients may begin to view healthcare through the lens of a service they are purchasing.

Gradually, the patient begins to resemble a consumer.

This shift does not occur intentionally. It emerges naturally when healthcare becomes intertwined with financial transactions. Patients who invest substantial resources into treatment often expect outcomes similar to those associated with other services in modern society.

They expect clarity, efficiency, accountability, and results.

When healthcare is experienced in this way, expectations can change. Patients may evaluate hospitals and doctors in terms of service quality, waiting times, technological sophistication, and overall treatment experience.

These expectations are understandable.

Illness places individuals and families in vulnerable positions, and the financial burden associated with treatment can amplify this vulnerability. When people pay significant amounts for healthcare services, they naturally expect transparency and value in return.

However, the consumer model introduces subtle tensions into the doctor–patient relationship.

In many services, consumers expect guaranteed results. If a product fails, it can be replaced or refunded. Medicine, however, operates under very different conditions. Biological systems are complex, and outcomes cannot always be predicted with certainty.

Even the best medical care cannot guarantee recovery in every case.

When patients approach healthcare as consumers, this uncertainty can lead to frustration. If treatment outcomes do not meet expectations, patients may interpret the situation as a failure of service rather than the natural unpredictability of medical science.

The consultation room begins to carry elements of transaction rather than partnership.

Doctors may also feel the effects of this shift. Physicians who once functioned primarily as professional advisors may now be perceived as service providers within a larger healthcare marketplace. Patients may expect detailed explanations, immediate availability, and measurable outcomes.

These expectations can place additional pressure on doctors.

Hospitals sometimes reinforce this consumer perspective through marketing and branding strategies. Healthcare institutions may advertise advanced technologies, premium facilities, or specialized treatment packages. Such messaging can unintentionally frame healthcare as a competitive marketplace.

Patients begin comparing hospitals the way they might compare other services.

While competition can drive improvements in quality and efficiency, it can also influence how people interpret the purpose of medicine. Healing may appear as a product delivered by institutions rather than a complex process involving cooperation between doctor and patient.

This transformation alters the emotional atmosphere of healthcare.

When patients see themselves primarily as consumers, they may approach consultations with expectations shaped by market logic. When doctors are viewed as service providers, their professional judgment may be evaluated through the standards applied to other industries.

The deeper relationship between doctor and patient risks becoming overshadowed.

Recognizing this shift is important because it reveals one of the central tensions of modern medicine. Healthcare must operate within economic systems to remain sustainable, yet the essence of medicine remains fundamentally human.

Doctors and patients must therefore navigate a delicate balance.

Patients deserve transparency, accountability, and respect for the financial sacrifices they make to access treatment. At the same time, medicine must remain grounded in professional judgment, scientific understanding, and the recognition that healing cannot always be reduced to a predictable transaction.

Maintaining this balance is one of the defining challenges of healthcare in the modern era.

9.5 — The Pharmaceutical and Technology Ecosystem

Modern medicine does not operate only through doctors and hospitals. Surrounding the clinical practice of healthcare is a vast ecosystem of industries that develop medicines, design medical devices, manufacture diagnostic technologies, and support the scientific research that drives medical progress.

This ecosystem has transformed the capabilities of modern medicine.

Pharmaceutical companies invest enormous resources into discovering and developing new drugs. The process begins with scientific research into the biological mechanisms of disease. Researchers identify molecules that may influence these processes and then test them through laboratory studies, animal models, and eventually clinical trials involving human participants.

This journey from discovery to approved medication can take many years.

Regulatory authorities carefully evaluate these medicines to ensure safety and effectiveness before they are made available to patients. Once approved, pharmaceutical companies must manufacture the drugs at scale, distribute them across healthcare systems, and monitor their effects through continued research.

The result is a constant stream of new treatments that improve the management of many diseases.

At the same time, technological innovation has reshaped how doctors diagnose and treat illness. Medical imaging technologies such as ultrasound, CT scans, and MRI machines allow physicians to see structures inside the body with remarkable clarity. Surgical tools have evolved from traditional instruments to minimally invasive techniques and robotic systems capable of performing delicate procedures.

Diagnostic laboratories now analyze biological samples with extraordinary precision.

These technological advances have saved countless lives and improved the quality of care available to patients around the world. Diseases that once required guesswork can now be diagnosed accurately. Treatments that were once impossible have become routine.

Medicine has advanced because of this powerful ecosystem.

However, this ecosystem also operates within economic realities.

Pharmaceutical companies and technology manufacturers invest large amounts of capital into research and development. Recovering these investments requires commercial models that allow companies to sustain operations and continue funding future innovation.

As a result, the development of medicines and technologies is closely connected with market dynamics.

Hospitals and healthcare institutions purchase diagnostic machines, surgical systems, and laboratory technologies from specialized manufacturers. Pharmaceutical companies promote new medicines to healthcare providers through educational programs, conferences, and scientific publications.

These interactions create a network of relationships between industry and medical practice.

Most of these relationships exist to support innovation and improve treatment options. Doctors depend on new medicines and technologies to provide better care to patients. Without scientific research and industrial development, many of the treatments available today would not exist.

Yet the presence of commercial incentives can also create ethical questions.

When companies market medicines or technologies aggressively, some observers worry that commercial interests might influence how treatments are promoted or adopted within healthcare systems. Doctors must therefore evaluate new products carefully, ensuring that clinical decisions remain guided by scientific evidence and patient welfare.

Medical professionals are trained to maintain this balance.

Clinical guidelines, peer-reviewed research, and regulatory oversight help ensure that new medicines and technologies are used appropriately. These mechanisms exist to protect patients and preserve the integrity of medical practice.

Nevertheless, the influence of the pharmaceutical and technology ecosystem remains significant.

Doctors operate within a landscape where scientific progress and commercial enterprise intersect. Hospitals rely on advanced technologies to provide modern care. Patients benefit from medicines and devices developed through years of research and investment.

Understanding this ecosystem helps explain how modern medicine functions.

Healthcare today is not shaped only by doctors and patients. It is supported by a vast network of scientific research, industrial development, and technological innovation. This network brings extraordinary benefits but also introduces economic forces that must be balanced carefully to preserve the fundamental purpose of medicine: healing human life.

9.6 — When Incentives Distort Decisions

Economic systems exist to sustain healthcare infrastructure, support innovation, and ensure that hospitals and industries can continue operating. In principle, these financial structures serve an important purpose. Without investment and organized funding, modern healthcare systems could not maintain the advanced technologies, trained personnel, and research capabilities that patients depend upon.

However, whenever financial incentives enter a system built on human care, the possibility of distortion also appears.

Most doctors enter medicine with the intention of practicing healing and applying scientific knowledge to improve lives. Yet when healthcare operates within complex economic frameworks, the environment surrounding medical decisions can sometimes influence how care is delivered.

These influences are often subtle rather than intentional.

For example, hospitals must maintain financial sustainability to continue operating. The infrastructure required for modern healthcare—diagnostic equipment, specialized staff, and intensive care units—requires constant funding. Institutions therefore develop financial models that allow them to recover operational costs.

Within such systems, certain procedures or services may generate more revenue than others.

Doctors working within these environments may encounter institutional expectations related to patient volume, diagnostic utilization, or treatment pathways. Even when these expectations are not explicitly stated, the organizational culture of an institution can influence how healthcare is structured.

This creates ethical tension for physicians.

Clinical judgment ideally focuses entirely on what is medically necessary for the patient. But when institutional incentives exist in the background, doctors may sometimes feel pressure—direct or indirect—to align their decisions with organizational priorities.

The challenge is rarely black and white.

In many cases, diagnostic tests or procedures that generate revenue are also medically appropriate. Advanced imaging, laboratory investigations, and specialized treatments often improve diagnostic accuracy and treatment outcomes.

Yet the boundary between necessity and excess can sometimes become blurred.

Debates about over-testing and over-treatment have emerged in many healthcare systems around the world. Some critics argue that financial incentives encourage excessive diagnostic procedures or treatments that may not always be essential. Others point out that defensive medicine and technological availability also contribute to this trend.

Doctors must navigate these debates carefully.

Most physicians rely on clinical guidelines, professional ethics, and personal judgment to determine what is appropriate for each patient. Their goal is to ensure that treatment decisions remain guided by medical necessity rather than financial opportunity.

However, the perception of financial influence can still affect how patients interpret medical advice.

When patients know that hospitals operate within economic systems, they may wonder whether certain recommendations are influenced by institutional incentives. Even when doctors act entirely in the patient's best interest, the surrounding financial structures can create doubt.

This perception can weaken trust.

Doctors themselves often feel uncomfortable when economic considerations appear to intersect with clinical decisions. Many physicians prefer to maintain a clear separation between the science of medicine and the financial structures that support healthcare institutions.

Maintaining this separation, however, is not always easy within large healthcare systems.

Recognizing the possibility of distorted incentives is important because it encourages healthcare systems to develop safeguards. Transparent policies, ethical guidelines, and regulatory oversight help ensure that patient welfare remains the central priority of medical practice.

Hospitals, professional associations, and governments all play roles in maintaining this balance.

The goal is not to eliminate economic structures from healthcare—such systems are necessary for sustaining modern medicine. Instead, the challenge is to ensure that financial incentives never overshadow the fundamental purpose of healthcare.

Medicine exists first to heal.

When economic systems support this purpose responsibly, they strengthen healthcare. But when incentives begin to influence decisions in ways that conflict with patient welfare, the integrity of medicine itself is placed at risk.

Maintaining this balance remains one of the most important responsibilities within modern healthcare systems.

9.7 — Restoring Balance Between Care and Commerce

Modern healthcare cannot exist without economic structures. Hospitals require funding to operate, technologies must be purchased and maintained, professionals must be trained and compensated, and research must be financed. These realities make it impossible to separate medicine entirely from economics.

The challenge, therefore, is not to eliminate the economic dimension of healthcare.

The challenge is to ensure that economic systems support the purpose of medicine rather than overshadow it.

Restoring balance between care and commerce begins with reaffirming the central role of patient welfare. Every healthcare system—whether public or private—must be designed around the principle that medical decisions should primarily serve the well-being of patients.

Economic sustainability should support this mission, not replace it.

Doctors play a crucial role in maintaining this balance. Physicians often stand at the point where clinical judgment meets institutional structure. Their professional ethics guide them to evaluate treatments based on medical necessity, evidence, and the individual needs of the patient.

When doctors remain committed to these principles, they act as safeguards within the system.

Professional integrity becomes especially important in environments where financial incentives exist. A doctor who prioritizes the patient's health over institutional pressure helps preserve the moral foundation of medicine.

Ethical leadership within healthcare institutions is equally important.

Hospital administrators and healthcare leaders must design policies that encourage responsible medical practice. Performance metrics, operational targets, and financial planning should align with patient-centered values rather than purely commercial outcomes.

Transparent systems can strengthen public trust.

When hospitals clearly communicate treatment costs, procedures, and clinical reasoning, patients are more likely to understand the decisions being made. Transparency reduces suspicion and allows patients to see that healthcare institutions are committed to fairness and accountability.

Governments and regulatory bodies also have a responsibility in maintaining balance.

Public policies can establish guidelines that prevent exploitative practices while ensuring that healthcare systems remain financially sustainable. Regulatory oversight helps ensure that medicines, technologies, and medical procedures meet ethical and scientific standards.

These frameworks create boundaries within which healthcare institutions operate.

Patients themselves contribute to this balance as well. When patients understand that medicine involves both scientific uncertainty and economic realities, they can engage more constructively with healthcare providers.

Expecting guaranteed outcomes from complex biological systems can place unrealistic pressure on doctors.

Recognizing that medicine is both a science and a human practice encourages more realistic expectations and healthier cooperation between patients and physicians.

The ultimate goal is not to return to a romanticized past where medicine existed outside economic systems. Such a world no longer exists. The scale and complexity of modern healthcare require organized financial structures.

Instead, the goal is to ensure that commerce remains the servant of care.

Economic systems should sustain hospitals, support innovation, and make treatments accessible. At the same time, they must never replace the fundamental purpose of medicine: the restoration of health and the protection of human life.

When this balance is maintained, healthcare systems can achieve both sustainability and integrity.

Doctors can practice medicine with confidence in their ethical responsibilities. Patients can seek care with trust in the intentions of those treating them. Institutions can operate effectively without losing sight of their human purpose.

In such an environment, medicine continues to advance without forgetting the reason it exists in the first place.

Medicine Beyond the Marketplace

Modern medicine stands at a remarkable point in human history. Scientific progress has given doctors tools that previous generations could scarcely imagine. Diseases that once devastated communities can now be prevented or treated. Complex surgeries restore lives. Diagnostic technologies reveal conditions with extraordinary precision.

Healthcare has become one of the most advanced achievements of modern civilization.

Yet alongside this progress, medicine has also become deeply intertwined with economic systems. Hospitals require large infrastructures, research requires enormous investment, and healthcare services operate within organized financial structures.

The healing profession now exists within a marketplace.

This transformation is neither entirely good nor entirely harmful. Economic systems have made it possible to build hospitals, develop life-saving medicines, and expand healthcare access to millions of people. Without financial organization and investment, many of the medical advances that define modern healthcare would not exist.

Commerce has enabled progress.

At the same time, the presence of economic incentives introduces a subtle risk. When healthcare becomes too closely aligned with market logic, the deeper purpose of medicine can begin to blur. Patients may start to feel like customers navigating a service industry rather than individuals seeking care in moments of vulnerability.

Doctors may feel that their professional judgment is evaluated through financial frameworks rather than clinical reasoning.

The consultation room begins to carry the weight of transactions.

But medicine cannot be reduced entirely to market principles.

A doctor cannot promise guaranteed outcomes the way a business promises products. Illness does not follow predictable patterns, and healing depends on biological processes that remain complex and uncertain. Even the most skilled physicians sometimes confront situations where science has limits.

This reality reminds us that medicine remains fundamentally human.

At its core, healthcare involves trust, responsibility, compassion, and the application of knowledge to relieve suffering. These qualities cannot be measured purely through financial metrics or institutional performance indicators.

They exist in the quiet space where a doctor listens carefully to a patient's fears.

The challenge for modern healthcare is therefore not to reject economic systems but to ensure that they remain aligned with the deeper mission of medicine. Hospitals must remain financially sustainable, industries must continue developing new treatments, and governments must design systems that support access to care.

But none of these structures should replace the human relationship at the center of healing.

When doctors remember that every case represents a human life, and when patients recognize that medicine involves both expertise and uncertainty, the balance between care and commerce becomes easier to maintain.

The marketplace may surround medicine, but it should never define it.

Because long before hospitals became institutions and healthcare became an industry, medicine began with a simple purpose: one human being helping another recover from illness.

Preserving that purpose remains the responsibility of everyone who participates in the modern healthcare system.

Chapter 10 — The Degree Without Depth

When Knowledge Becomes Certification

The journey to becoming a doctor has traditionally been one of the most demanding paths in professional education. It requires years of disciplined study, continuous observation, and exposure to real human suffering. Medical training is not only about acquiring information; it is about developing judgment, responsibility, and the ability to act under uncertainty.

A medical degree, therefore, has always carried a deeper meaning.

It represents not just academic success, but a transformation of the individual. A student enters medical education with curiosity and ambition, but is expected to emerge with the capacity to make decisions that affect human life. The white coat becomes a symbol of this transformation—a visible reminder that knowledge must be applied with care and responsibility.

But when systems expand rapidly, the meaning of this symbol can begin to shift.

In many parts of the world, the demand for healthcare professionals has increased significantly. Populations are growing, healthcare systems are expanding, and the need for doctors continues to rise. To meet this demand, the number of medical institutions has increased, and access to medical education has widened.

This expansion has brought both opportunity and risk.

Opportunity, because more individuals can now pursue careers in medicine, increasing the availability of healthcare services. Risk, because when systems grow quickly, maintaining consistent standards becomes more challenging.

In such environments, a subtle shift can occur.

The medical degree, which once reflected deep understanding and rigorous training, may begin to appear as a certification—a document that signifies completion of a program rather than mastery of a discipline. When this happens, the focus can move from learning to qualifying.

Students may begin to see the degree as the goal rather than the knowledge it represents.

This transformation is not always visible from the outside. A doctor holds the same title, wears the same white coat, and occupies the same position within society. Patients continue to place trust in the symbol of the profession.

Yet the depth behind that symbol may vary.

Medicine is not a field where surface-level understanding is sufficient. Diagnosing illness requires the ability to interpret subtle patterns in symptoms. Treating patients involves balancing multiple factors—biological, psychological, and social. Clinical decisions often must be made under conditions of uncertainty.

Such responsibilities demand more than certification.

They require deep understanding, critical thinking, and the ability to connect knowledge with real-world situations. When training systems fail to cultivate these qualities consistently, the gap between degree and competence can widen.

This gap carries consequences.

For patients, it may appear as inconsistent quality of care. For the medical profession, it may lead to questions about credibility and trust. For doctors themselves, it can create internal challenges when they face situations that require skills beyond what their training has fully developed.

Recognizing this issue is not about questioning the dedication of individual doctors.

Many physicians work tirelessly to build their knowledge and skills despite systemic challenges. The concern lies in the structures that produce medical professionals and whether those structures consistently ensure the depth required for such a critical profession.

Because in medicine, a degree is not merely a qualification.

It is a responsibility carried into every consultation, every diagnosis, and every decision that affects human life.

10.1 — The Long Journey to Becoming a Doctor

Becoming a doctor has traditionally been one of the most demanding intellectual and emotional journeys in professional life. It is not a path defined by a single examination or a limited period of study. It is a prolonged process that requires sustained discipline, deep curiosity, and the ability to remain committed even under pressure.

The journey often begins long before medical college.

Students who aspire to enter medicine must first compete in highly selective entrance examinations. These exams test not only academic knowledge but also the ability to perform under intense competition. For many, this phase involves years of preparation, long study hours, and significant personal sacrifice.

Earning a seat in a medical college is therefore itself a major achievement.

Once admitted, the nature of learning changes fundamentally. Medical education is not limited to memorizing facts. Students must understand the structure and function of the human body in detail—anatomy, physiology, biochemistry, and later, pathology, pharmacology, and clinical medicine.

Each subject builds upon the previous one.

Understanding anatomy requires visualization of complex structures. Physiology demands comprehension of dynamic processes within the body. Pharmacology involves understanding how drugs interact with biological systems. These subjects are not isolated; they form an interconnected framework that students must learn to integrate.

This integration is essential for clinical practice.

As students progress, they move from classrooms into clinical environments. Hospitals become learning spaces where theoretical knowledge meets real human situations. Students observe patients, assist senior doctors, and gradually begin to understand how symptoms, history, and physical examination combine to form a diagnosis.

This stage transforms learning into experience.

Clinical training exposes students to the unpredictability of medicine. No two patients present exactly the same way, even with similar conditions. Students learn to interpret variations, to recognize patterns, and to remain cautious when certainty is not possible.

They begin to understand that medicine is not only a science but also an art of judgment.

Mentorship plays a crucial role in this process. Senior doctors guide students through complex cases, demonstrating how to approach diagnosis and treatment. These interactions shape not only knowledge but also professional behavior—how to communicate with patients, how to handle uncertainty, and how to make decisions responsibly.

This mentorship helps bridge the gap between theory and practice.

The journey is also emotionally demanding.

Medical students and young doctors encounter suffering, pain, and sometimes loss. These experiences require them to develop emotional resilience while maintaining compassion. Balancing empathy with professional composure becomes an essential part of their training.

This emotional dimension is often as challenging as the intellectual one.

Even after formal education, learning does not end. Medicine evolves continuously, and doctors must keep updating their knowledge throughout their careers. New research, treatments, and technologies require ongoing study and adaptation.

The profession demands lifelong learning.

This long journey explains why society places such trust in doctors. The medical degree is not simply a certificate of academic completion; it represents years of rigorous preparation, practical exposure, and personal development.

It signifies readiness to take responsibility for human health.

However, this ideal journey depends on the quality and integrity of the educational system that supports it. When every stage of this process is conducted with seriousness and depth, the result is a doctor capable of making thoughtful and responsible decisions.

When any part of this journey is weakened, the depth behind the degree may also be affected.

Understanding the traditional path to becoming a doctor helps highlight what is at stake when medical education systems face challenges. Because in medicine, the journey itself shapes the quality of the professional who eventually stands before the patient.

10.2 — The Expansion of Medical Education

Over the past few decades, healthcare systems around the world have undergone rapid expansion. Populations have grown, life expectancy has increased, and the demand for medical services has risen significantly. Governments and private sectors alike have recognized the need for more doctors to meet this growing demand.

This necessity has led to a major expansion in medical education.

New medical colleges have been established, existing institutions have increased their intake capacity, and opportunities to pursue medical training have become more widely available. In countries like India, this expansion has been particularly visible, with a significant rise in both public and private medical institutions.

At one level, this expansion represents progress.

More medical colleges mean more doctors, which can improve access to healthcare services, especially in regions where medical professionals were previously scarce. Increased availability of education also allows more students to pursue careers in medicine, contributing to the overall development of healthcare systems.

However, rapid expansion introduces its own challenges.

Medical education is not simply about increasing the number of seats. It requires maintaining high standards of teaching, ensuring access to quality clinical exposure, and providing experienced faculty who can guide students effectively.

When the number of institutions grows faster than the availability of these resources, maintaining consistency becomes difficult.

Some medical colleges may struggle to provide adequate clinical exposure to students. Hospitals attached to educational institutions may not have sufficient patient inflow to offer diverse learning experiences. Faculty shortages can limit the depth of teaching, and infrastructure may not always match the standards required for comprehensive training.

These gaps can affect the learning process.

In such environments, students may complete their education with varying levels of practical experience. While they may have studied the required subjects, their exposure to real-world clinical situations might be limited.

This creates differences in how well prepared graduates are for independent medical practice.

The expansion of private medical colleges has also introduced a new dimension.

Private institutions often operate within financial frameworks that require sustainability through fees and investments. While many private colleges maintain high standards, the economic model of such institutions can sometimes influence how education is structured.

The pressure to accommodate more students may compete with the need to maintain rigorous training conditions.

At the same time, the increasing demand for medical seats reflects the aspirations of students and families. Medicine continues to be seen as a prestigious and stable profession, attracting large numbers of applicants each year.

This demand creates competition not only for entry into medical colleges but also for the resources required to train future doctors effectively.

Balancing quantity and quality becomes the central challenge.

Healthcare systems need more doctors, but they also need doctors who are well trained, capable, and responsible. Expanding the number of institutions without ensuring consistent standards risks creating variation in the depth of medical education.

This variation can have long-term implications.

When patients interact with doctors, they do not distinguish between institutions or training pathways. They place trust in the profession as a whole. If educational standards vary widely, that trust can be affected.

Understanding the expansion of medical education is therefore essential.

It highlights the tension between the need to increase access to medical training and the responsibility to maintain the depth and rigor that the profession demands. The future of healthcare depends not only on the number of doctors available but also on the quality of their preparation.

Because in medicine, expansion without depth can create challenges that extend far beyond the classroom.

10.3 — When Admission Becomes Transactional

One of the most sensitive and consequential shifts in medical education occurs when the process of admission begins to move away from merit and toward financial capability. Medicine has traditionally been a field where entry is determined by rigorous competition, demanding both intellectual ability and sustained effort.

This merit-based pathway ensures that those who enter the profession are prepared for the complexity and responsibility it demands.

However, in systems where medical education becomes expensive and seats are limited, a parallel pathway can emerge—one influenced by financial transactions. High tuition fees, management quotas, and donation-based admissions in some institutions introduce the possibility that entry into medical education may not always reflect academic merit alone.

When this happens, the perception of medicine begins to shift.

Students who secure admission primarily through financial means may still complete the same curriculum and obtain the same degree. On paper, their qualifications appear identical to those who entered through competitive merit-based processes.

But the journey that leads to that degree may differ significantly.

Medical education requires not only access to classrooms but also the capacity to engage deeply with the material. Students must develop critical thinking, clinical reasoning, and the discipline to handle demanding workloads. When admission is driven by merit, it often reflects a student's readiness for this level of engagement.

When admission becomes transactional, this readiness cannot always be assumed.

This does not mean that every student entering through financial pathways lacks capability or commitment. Many may work hard and develop strong clinical skills over time. However, the system itself introduces variability in the baseline preparedness of students entering medical training.

This variability can influence the learning environment.

In classrooms and clinical settings, differences in foundational knowledge and motivation may become visible. Faculty may need to adapt teaching methods to accommodate varying levels of understanding. The pace of learning can be affected, and the overall depth of training may vary across institutions.

Over time, these differences can extend into professional practice.

Patients, however, do not see the admission pathway of the doctor they consult. They trust the degree as a symbol of competence and responsibility. When the public begins to perceive that entry into medicine can be influenced by financial means, questions naturally arise about the uniformity of training and the reliability of professional standards.

Trust becomes vulnerable.

This issue also creates ethical tension within the system. Students who enter through highly competitive merit-based processes may feel that the integrity of the profession is being diluted. Those who enter through financial pathways may face internal pressure to prove their capability in environments where expectations are already high.

The profession becomes internally divided in subtle ways.

Institutions themselves face difficult choices. Private medical colleges require financial sustainability, and tuition fees form a major part of their operational model. Balancing this financial necessity with the responsibility to maintain rigorous admission standards is a complex challenge.

Without careful regulation, the system can drift toward imbalance.

The deeper concern lies not only in individual cases but in the message that such systems send to society. If medicine is perceived as a profession that can be accessed through financial means rather than earned through merit and dedication, the symbolic value of the medical degree begins to weaken.

And with it, the trust associated with the profession.

Addressing this issue requires acknowledging that admission processes shape the future of healthcare. The quality of doctors is influenced not only by what they learn during training but also by the standards applied when they enter the system.

Because in medicine, the journey begins long before the degree is awarded—and the integrity of that journey determines the depth behind the profession itself.

10.4 — The Difference Between Passing Exams and Understanding Medicine

Medical education, like all structured learning systems, relies on examinations to assess progress. Students are tested on their knowledge of anatomy, physiology, pathology, pharmacology, and clinical subjects. These exams serve an important purpose—they ensure that students have engaged with the required material and reached a certain level of academic competence.

But passing examinations is not the same as understanding medicine.

Examinations often reward the ability to recall information, recognize patterns, and reproduce learned concepts within a limited time. Students prepare by studying textbooks, attending lectures, and practicing past questions. With discipline and effort, many can successfully navigate these assessments.

However, real medical practice demands something deeper.

A patient does not present with a question paper. Symptoms are rarely organized in neat categories. A person may arrive with multiple complaints, incomplete information, or conditions that do not fit textbook descriptions perfectly.

The doctor must interpret, connect, and decide.

This requires clinical understanding—the ability to apply knowledge to real situations. It involves recognizing patterns in symptoms, understanding how different systems of the body interact, and evaluating probabilities when certainty is not possible.

Clinical understanding cannot be developed through memorization alone.

It grows through observation, experience, and guided practice. Students must see patients, listen to histories, perform examinations, and watch how experienced doctors approach complex cases. They must learn not only *what* to think but *how* to think.

This is where the role of mentorship becomes critical.

Senior doctors demonstrate how to approach uncertainty, how to balance multiple possibilities, and how to make decisions responsibly. They teach students how to prioritize information, how to communicate with patients, and how to remain composed under pressure.

These lessons are rarely captured fully in textbooks or exams.

The distinction between passing exams and understanding medicine becomes especially important in clinical decision-making. A student may know the theoretical features of a disease but may struggle to recognize it when presented in an atypical form. Another may understand pharmacological principles but may find it difficult to adjust treatment for a patient with multiple conditions.

Real-world medicine requires integration of knowledge.

It also demands judgment. Doctors must decide when to order tests, when to begin treatment, when to wait and observe, and when to seek additional opinions. These decisions often involve balancing risks and benefits under conditions of uncertainty.

Such judgment develops over time through experience and reflection.

When medical education focuses too heavily on examination performance, there is a risk that students may prioritize short-term success over long-term understanding. They may learn to pass tests efficiently without fully developing the depth required for clinical practice.

The degree is obtained, but the learning may remain incomplete.

Patients, however, depend on more than academic achievement. They rely on the doctor's ability to interpret their condition accurately and respond appropriately. This expectation requires a level of understanding that goes beyond what examinations alone can measure.

Recognizing this difference is essential for maintaining the integrity of medical education.

Examinations should serve as checkpoints, not endpoints. They should support learning rather than replace it. True medical competence emerges when knowledge, experience, and judgment come together in the service of patient care.

Because in medicine, understanding is not demonstrated by passing an exam—it is demonstrated in the decisions made when a human life depends on them.

10.5 — The Consequences for Patients and Society

When the depth of medical education is compromised—even subtly—the consequences do not remain confined to classrooms or institutions. They extend outward, directly affecting patients, families, and the broader trust that society places in the medical profession.

Medicine is one of the few fields where the margin for error is extremely narrow.

A small lapse in understanding can lead to a missed diagnosis. An incomplete grasp of pharmacology can result in incorrect medication or dosage. A lack of clinical judgment can delay critical decisions. In many professions, mistakes can be corrected over time; in medicine, delays or errors can have immediate and irreversible effects.

For patients, these consequences are deeply personal.

They approach doctors at moments of vulnerability—when they are in pain, uncertain, or fearful. They trust that the person in front of them has the knowledge and capability to guide them through that situation. This trust is not based on personal verification of competence but on the belief that the system producing doctors ensures a certain standard.

When that standard varies, the experience of care can become inconsistent.

One patient may receive accurate diagnosis and effective treatment, while another with a similar condition may encounter delays, confusion, or inappropriate interventions. These variations are not always visible at a systemic level, but they are deeply felt at the individual level.

Over time, such experiences shape public perception.

When patients or their families encounter poor outcomes that they attribute to inadequate medical judgment, confidence in the profession begins to weaken. Stories circulate, experiences are shared, and a general sense of skepticism can develop.

Trust, once affected, is difficult to rebuild.

This erosion of trust has broader implications for society. Healthcare systems rely heavily on cooperation between doctors and patients. Treatment plans require adherence, follow-ups depend on patient participation, and preventive care depends on public confidence in medical advice.

When trust declines, this cooperation weakens.

Patients may begin to question medical recommendations, delay seeking treatment, or rely on alternative sources of information that may not always be reliable. Communication between doctors and patients can become strained, with both sides approaching interactions defensively.

The relationship shifts from collaboration to negotiation.

The consequences also extend to the medical profession itself. Doctors who are well trained and committed to their work may find themselves operating in an environment where their credibility is questioned due to the actions or perceived shortcomings of others.

The profession carries collective responsibility.

This can create frustration and additional pressure for practitioners who must not only provide care but also rebuild trust in each interaction. It adds a layer of complexity to an already demanding profession.

At a systemic level, the impact can be even more significant.

Healthcare policies, legal frameworks, and regulatory measures may become more stringent in response to declining trust. Increased oversight, while necessary in some cases, can also introduce additional administrative burdens for doctors, affecting their ability to focus on patient care.

The system becomes more controlled, but not necessarily more effective.

Understanding these consequences highlights the importance of maintaining depth in medical education. The issue is not limited to individual competence; it affects the entire ecosystem of healthcare.

Because in medicine, the quality of training is directly linked to the quality of care—and the quality of care shapes the trust that sustains the entire system.

10.6 — The Responsibility of Regulatory Bodies

In a profession as critical as medicine, individual effort alone cannot guarantee consistent standards. Even the most dedicated students and committed teachers operate within systems that shape their opportunities, exposure, and evaluation. This is where regulatory bodies play a central role.

They are the custodians of quality.

Regulatory institutions are responsible for ensuring that medical education maintains its depth, rigor, and integrity across all institutions. Their role is not merely administrative; it is foundational. They define standards, approve institutions, monitor performance, and ensure that the pathway from student to doctor remains credible.

Without effective regulation, variation becomes inevitable.

As medical education expands, differences in infrastructure, faculty strength, and clinical exposure naturally emerge. Some institutions may maintain high standards, while others may struggle. Regulatory bodies are expected to identify these gaps and ensure that minimum benchmarks are consistently met.

This responsibility is both preventive and corrective.

Preventive, in the sense that institutions must meet defined criteria before they are allowed to function. Corrective, in the sense that ongoing monitoring must identify deviations and enforce improvements where necessary. Accreditation, inspections, and periodic evaluations are tools designed to maintain this balance.

But regulation must go beyond formality.

If oversight becomes limited to documentation and periodic inspections, it risks missing the deeper realities of medical training. A college may meet formal requirements on paper while still lacking the quality of teaching, mentorship, or clinical exposure needed for effective learning.

True regulation requires understanding the ground reality.

This includes evaluating not just infrastructure, but also the quality of teaching, the engagement of faculty, and the actual learning experience of students. It requires feedback systems that capture what happens inside classrooms and hospitals, not just what is reported in official records.

The focus must remain on outcomes, not just processes.

Another critical responsibility of regulatory bodies lies in maintaining the integrity of admissions. Transparent, merit-based selection processes are essential to ensure that students entering medical education are prepared for the demands of the profession.

When admission standards are compromised, the entire system is affected.

Regulators must therefore design and enforce frameworks that minimize the influence of financial transactions in admission processes. This is not only about fairness but also about ensuring that the future workforce of healthcare is competent and reliable.

Licensing and competency evaluation also fall within their scope.

Before a medical graduate begins independent practice, there must be mechanisms to assess whether they possess the required knowledge and clinical skills. Standardized examinations, internships, and supervised practice periods serve as critical checkpoints in this transition.

These checkpoints protect patients.

Regulation must also extend into professional life. Continuous medical education, periodic re-certification, and ethical guidelines ensure that doctors remain updated and accountable throughout their careers.

Medicine evolves, and regulation must evolve with it.

At the same time, regulatory bodies face their own challenges. Balancing strict oversight with practical feasibility, managing large numbers of institutions, and adapting to changing healthcare needs require careful planning and execution.

Over-regulation can create rigidity, while under-regulation can lead to decline in standards.

The goal is to maintain equilibrium.

Effective regulation does not restrict the growth of medical education; it strengthens it. It ensures that expansion does not come at the cost of quality, and that every degree awarded carries a consistent level of credibility.

Because in medicine, regulation is not about control—it is about safeguarding the trust that society places in the profession.

And that trust begins long before a doctor meets a patient.

10.7 — Restoring Depth in Medical Training

If the concern is that medical education risks becoming shallow in parts of the system, then the response cannot be cosmetic. It must be structural, intentional, and sustained. Restoring depth is not about adding more content—it is about redefining how learning happens, how competence is built, and how responsibility is internalized.

The first step is to realign the purpose of medical education.

The goal is not to produce degree holders; it is to produce decision-makers. Doctors are not evaluated by how much they remember, but by how effectively they interpret, prioritize, and act under uncertainty. Training systems must therefore shift focus from information accumulation to clinical thinking.

This requires redesigning how students engage with knowledge.

Conceptual clarity must take precedence over rote learning. Instead of treating subjects as isolated silos, education must emphasize integration—how physiology connects with pathology, how pharmacology influences treatment decisions, and how clinical presentation reflects underlying mechanisms.

Students must learn to connect, not just collect.

Clinical exposure must also become more meaningful.

Hospitals should not be passive observation spaces where students merely watch senior doctors work. They must become active learning environments where students participate, ask questions, and gradually take responsibility under supervision. Exposure to diverse cases, including common and complex conditions, is essential for developing clinical judgment.

Learning must move from seeing to doing.

Mentorship is the backbone of this transformation.

Experienced doctors must not only treat patients but also actively shape the next generation. Teaching should not be limited to formal lectures; it should happen during rounds, case discussions, and real-time decision-making. Students learn deeply when they see how experienced clinicians think, not just what they know.

This transfer of thinking is what creates depth.

Assessment systems must also evolve.

Examinations should test understanding, reasoning, and application rather than memorization. Case-based evaluations, problem-solving scenarios, and practical assessments can better reflect a student's readiness for clinical practice. When assessments reward depth, students naturally align their learning toward it.

Evaluation must reflect reality.

Admissions processes need to reinforce merit and preparedness.

Ensuring that students entering medical education have the intellectual foundation and motivation required for the profession is critical. Transparent and fair selection mechanisms reduce variability at the entry point and create a stronger baseline for training.

The journey begins with the right foundation.

At a systemic level, institutions must be held accountable for outcomes.

It is not enough for colleges to demonstrate infrastructure and faculty numbers. They must be evaluated based on the competence of their graduates, the quality of their clinical training, and the feedback from students and patients. Continuous monitoring and improvement mechanisms are essential.

Quality must be measurable.

Technology can support this process but should not replace core learning.

Digital tools, simulations, and online resources can enhance understanding, but they cannot substitute real patient interaction. Medicine remains a human-centered field, and training must reflect this reality.

Technology should assist, not replace experience.

Finally, the culture of medical education must reinforce responsibility.

Students must understand from the beginning that a medical degree carries weight beyond personal achievement. It represents a commitment to society. Every diagnosis, every prescription, and every decision affects real lives.

This awareness must be cultivated early and consistently.

Restoring depth in medical training is not a single reform—it is a continuous process. It requires alignment between institutions, regulators, teachers, and students. It demands clarity of purpose and consistency of execution.

Because in medicine, depth is not optional.

It is the difference between treating a disease and truly caring for a human life.

The Meaning of the White Coat

At the end of this discussion lies a simple but uncomfortable question:

What does the white coat truly represent today?

To the public, it still carries a powerful image—knowledge, authority, trust, and safety. When a patient walks into a clinic or hospital, the white coat signals reassurance. It tells them that the person in front of them is capable, trained, and ready to help.

But symbols are only as strong as the reality behind them.

The white coat was never meant to be a decoration or a uniform of status. It emerged as a marker of responsibility—a visible reminder that the person wearing it has committed to a discipline that deals directly with human life. It signifies not only knowledge, but restraint, judgment, and accountability.

It is not worn for recognition. It is worn for responsibility.

When a doctor puts on the white coat, they step into a role that demands more than technical competence. They are expected to make decisions in uncertainty, to act when outcomes are not guaranteed, and to carry the consequences of those decisions.

No other profession combines knowledge, risk, and trust in quite the same way.

This is why the depth behind the degree matters so profoundly.

If the white coat becomes disconnected from the rigor of training, the seriousness of preparation, and the weight of responsibility, it risks becoming a symbol without substance. The appearance remains intact, but the meaning begins to fade.

And when meaning fades, trust follows.

Patients do not evaluate doctors through academic transcripts or institutional rankings. They experience the profession through interactions—through the clarity of explanation, the confidence of diagnosis, the appropriateness of treatment, and the sense of being understood.

The white coat is validated in these moments.

For doctors themselves, the white coat can also become a mirror.

It reflects not only what they have achieved, but what is expected of them. It asks a quiet question each day: *Is the knowledge I carry deep enough for the decisions I must make?* This question is not meant to create doubt, but to sustain awareness.

Because awareness maintains depth.

Restoring and preserving the meaning of the white coat does not depend on a single reform or regulation. It depends on a continuous alignment—between education and practice, between knowledge and action, between profession and purpose.

It depends on whether the system consistently produces doctors who understand the weight of what they carry.

In a world where healthcare continues to evolve, where systems grow more complex and pressures increase, the white coat must remain anchored to its original intent.

Not as a symbol of superiority, but as a commitment to service grounded in competence.

Because long after degrees are awarded and systems expand, what remains constant is the moment when a patient looks at a doctor and places trust in that white coat.

And that moment demands depth.

Chapter 11 — Society's Unrealistic Expectations

The Doctor as Everything

At some point, without formal agreement or conscious design, society began to expect more from doctors than any single profession can realistically deliver.

A doctor is no longer seen only as someone who diagnoses and treats illness.

They are expected to be precise like a scientist, compassionate like a counselor, available like a service provider, efficient like a manager, and ethical like a moral guide. In moments of crisis, they are expected to provide certainty where none exists, reassurance when outcomes are unclear, and solutions even when medicine itself has limits.

The expectation quietly expands with every interaction.

When a patient enters a clinic, they are not just bringing symptoms. They are bringing fear, confusion, financial concerns, and often a deep need for clarity. The doctor becomes the focal point for all of this. Every question, every doubt, every decision seems to converge at that one point—the person in the white coat.

The doctor becomes the system in the eyes of the patient.

This concentration of expectation is understandable.

Medicine deals with life, and when life feels threatened, people naturally look for someone who can take control of the situation. They want answers, direction, and assurance. They want someone who appears to know what is happening and what will happen next.

But this is where reality begins to diverge from expectation.

Medicine, despite all its progress, is not a domain of absolute certainty. It operates within probabilities, patterns, and evolving understanding. Even the most experienced doctors encounter cases where outcomes are unpredictable, responses vary, and decisions must be made with incomplete information.

Yet the expectation of certainty remains.

Patients often assume that a correct diagnosis should always be immediate, that treatment should always be effective, and that recovery should follow a predictable path. When these expectations are not met, the gap between what is expected and what is possible becomes visible.

And that gap creates tension.

At the same time, the role of the doctor has expanded beyond clinical care. Documentation requirements, administrative responsibilities, legal awareness, and communication demands have all increased. A doctor is now expected to manage not only the medical condition but also the process surrounding it.

The profession becomes multidimensional.

What makes this situation particularly complex is that these expectations are rarely expressed explicitly. They exist silently, embedded in how society perceives the profession. Doctors are expected to carry this weight naturally, without acknowledgment, as if it is an inherent part of their role.

The expectation becomes invisible—but not lighter.

For doctors, this creates a constant balancing act. They must navigate between what they know, what they can do, and what is expected of them. They must communicate uncertainty without reducing confidence, show empathy without losing objectivity, and make decisions under pressure while being aware of their consequences.

This balance is not easy to maintain.

Understanding this dynamic is essential, not to reduce expectations, but to make them realistic. Because when expectations exceed the nature of the profession, even sincere efforts can appear insufficient.

And when that happens, both the doctor and the patient feel the strain of a system where the role has quietly become larger than the individual who carries it.

11.1 — The Historical Image of the Doctor

Long before modern hospitals, advanced diagnostics, and complex healthcare systems existed, the figure of the doctor occupied a unique place in society. In many cultures, the healer was not just a practitioner of medicine but a figure of wisdom, authority, and reassurance.

The doctor was seen as someone who understood life more deeply than others.

This perception did not emerge from science alone. It was shaped by history, tradition, and human psychology. In earlier times, when medical knowledge was limited and diseases were poorly understood, the act of healing carried a certain mystique. Those who could relieve pain, treat illness, or even offer hope in uncertain situations were naturally elevated in social status.

The healer became a symbol of control in an uncontrollable world.

As medical science evolved, this image did not disappear—it strengthened. The discovery of antibiotics, the development of surgical techniques, and the ability to manage previously fatal conditions reinforced the belief that doctors possessed extraordinary capability.

Each medical breakthrough added to the aura of certainty.

Society began to associate doctors with solutions. Illness was no longer seen as an inevitable fate but as a problem that could be addressed, managed, or cured. The doctor became the central figure in this transformation—a professional who could intervene, correct, and restore.

This created a powerful narrative.

Over generations, this narrative shaped expectations. Families taught their children to trust doctors without question. Communities looked to them not only for treatment but also for guidance. In many cases, doctors were consulted not just for medical issues but for decisions related to life, health, and well-being.

Their role extended beyond medicine.

Respect for doctors became deeply embedded in cultural thinking. The white coat symbolized authority and knowledge, and the doctor's word carried weight. This respect was well deserved, built on years of rigorous training and the critical role doctors played in society.

But respect gradually merged with expectation.

As the image of the doctor evolved into that of a near-infallible figure, the distinction between expertise and perfection began to blur. The public perception shifted subtly—from seeing doctors as highly skilled professionals to expecting them to have answers for every situation.

The doctor became more than human in the eyes of society.

This historical buildup of trust and reverence created a foundation that continues to influence how doctors are perceived today. Even in a world where information is widely available and medical knowledge is understood to be evolving, the expectation of certainty persists.

The legacy of the past shapes the expectations of the present.

It is important to recognize that this perception was not created with negative intent. It emerged from genuine trust, gratitude, and the visible impact of medical progress. Doctors earned their position through dedication and contribution.

But the expectations that grew alongside this respect have become increasingly complex.

Understanding the historical image of the doctor helps explain why society continues to expect so much from the profession. It also highlights the need to differentiate between respect for expertise and the assumption of perfection.

Because while doctors have always been central to healing, they have never been beyond the limits of human capability.

11.2 — The Rise of Medical Expectations in the Modern Era

If the historical image of the doctor created the foundation of trust, modern medicine has amplified expectations to an entirely new level.

Advancements in science have transformed what is possible.

Diseases that once led to certain death are now treatable. Surgeries that were unimaginable a century ago are now routine. Diagnostic tools can detect conditions at early stages with remarkable accuracy. Intensive care units sustain life in situations that would have been fatal in the past.

Each advancement has reinforced a powerful belief:

Medicine can solve almost anything.

This belief, while rooted in real progress, has gradually shifted public expectations from hope to certainty. What was once considered exceptional has now become expected. A successful surgery is no longer seen as an achievement—it is assumed. A recovery is not appreciated as a probability—it is expected as an outcome.

Success has become the baseline.

At the same time, the visibility of medical success has increased dramatically. Media, digital platforms, and social narratives frequently highlight breakthrough treatments, miraculous recoveries, and cutting-edge procedures. These stories, while inspiring, create a selective perception of medicine.

They showcase what is possible, not what is typical.

Patients and families often approach healthcare with these narratives in mind. They expect rapid diagnosis, immediate intervention, and predictable recovery. The uncertainty that still exists within medicine is rarely part of this expectation.

But uncertainty remains central to medical practice.

Not every disease behaves predictably. Not every treatment works the same way for every patient. Biological systems are complex, and outcomes are influenced by multiple factors—genetics, environment, timing, and response to treatment.

Medicine operates within probabilities, not guarantees.

However, modern systems have reduced tolerance for this uncertainty. In many other domains—technology, services, consumer products—outcomes are standardized and predictable. This mindset has begun to influence how people perceive healthcare as well.

The expectation of precision becomes the expectation of perfection.

Patients may assume that if technology is advanced, then errors should not occur. If information is available, then diagnosis should be immediate. If treatment exists, then recovery should follow.

The complexity of medicine becomes simplified in perception.

This shift also affects how outcomes are interpreted. When treatment is successful, it aligns with expectation. When it is not, it is often perceived as failure—sometimes of the doctor, sometimes of the system, and sometimes of both.

The space for acceptance narrows.

Another factor contributing to rising expectations is access to information. Patients today are more informed than ever before.

They research symptoms, read about treatments, and explore multiple perspectives before consulting a doctor.

This awareness is valuable, but it can also create fixed expectations.

Patients may arrive with preconceived ideas about diagnosis or treatment, expecting confirmation rather than evaluation. When medical judgment differs from their expectation, it can lead to confusion or dissatisfaction.

The consultation becomes a negotiation rather than a process of discovery.

Doctors, therefore, operate in an environment where expectations are shaped not only by medical reality but also by perception, information, and societal narratives.

The gap between what medicine can do and what society expects it to do continues to widen.

Understanding this rise in expectations is essential—not to diminish the value of medical progress, but to place it in context. Modern medicine has achieved extraordinary advancements, but it has not eliminated uncertainty.

And as long as uncertainty exists, expectations must remain aligned with reality.

Because when expectations exceed the nature of the system, even the best outcomes may fail to satisfy—and the profession begins to carry a burden that no level of advancement can fully resolve.

11.3 — The Doctor as a Multirole Professional

In today's healthcare environment, the role of a doctor has expanded far beyond clinical expertise. Treating disease is no longer the only expectation. A doctor is now required to operate across multiple domains simultaneously—often within the same consultation.

The profession has become multidimensional.

At the core remains the clinical role. A doctor must diagnose, interpret symptoms, decide on investigations, and recommend treatment. This alone demands years of training, continuous learning, and the ability to make decisions under uncertainty.

But this is only one part of the role.

Patients today expect communication that is clear, detailed, and reassuring. They want to understand not only *what* is happening but *why* it is happening and *what will happen next*. The doctor must therefore become a communicator—translating complex medical information into language that is understandable and meaningful.

Clarity becomes part of care.

At the same time, emotional support is often expected. Patients and their families arrive with anxiety, fear, and sometimes distress. They look to the doctor not only for treatment but also for reassurance. In many cases, the doctor becomes an informal counselor—absorbing emotions while maintaining professional composure.

Empathy becomes an operational requirement.

Beyond this, administrative responsibilities have increased significantly. Documentation, prescriptions, reports, consent forms, insurance-related paperwork, and compliance with institutional protocols consume a considerable portion of a doctor's time.

The doctor becomes part of a system that requires process management.

Legal awareness has also become essential. Medical practice now operates within a framework where decisions may be scrutinized in legal contexts. Doctors must be careful not only about what they do, but also how they document and communicate it.

Every decision carries legal visibility.

In institutional settings, especially in large hospitals, doctors may also be required to align with organizational structures. This can include coordinating with departments, following protocols, managing time slots, and sometimes working within performance expectations related to patient flow or service delivery.

The clinical role intersects with operational realities.

In certain cases, doctors are also expected to guide patients on financial aspects—suggesting treatment options while being aware of cost implications. This adds another layer of complexity, where clinical decisions intersect with affordability and accessibility.

Medicine meets economics at the point of decision.

All these roles—clinician, communicator, counselor, administrator, and decision-maker—converge within the same individual. And often, they must be performed simultaneously, without clear boundaries separating them.

The expectation is seamless performance.

What makes this particularly challenging is that each of these roles requires a different skill set. Clinical expertise demands scientific understanding. Communication requires clarity and patience. Emotional support requires empathy. Administration requires organization. Legal awareness requires caution.

The doctor must switch between these modes continuously.

This multiplicity of roles is rarely acknowledged explicitly by society. Patients interact with doctors expecting all these functions to be performed naturally, as if they are inherent to the profession.

The complexity remains invisible, but the expectation remains constant.

For doctors, this creates a continuous cognitive and emotional load. They must not only treat the patient but also manage the interaction, document the process, consider legal implications, and navigate institutional frameworks—all within limited time.

The consultation becomes a compressed system of multiple responsibilities.

Understanding the doctor as a multirole professional is essential to appreciating the demands of modern medical practice. It highlights that the challenge is not only in diagnosing and treating disease but in managing the entire ecosystem that surrounds that process.

Because in today's world, a doctor is no longer just a medical expert.

They are a node where science, emotion, system, and society intersect—and that intersection carries a weight that is often underestimated.

11.4 — The Emotional Projection of Patients and Families

When a patient walks into a clinic or hospital, they rarely come alone—not just physically, but emotionally. Along with the symptoms, they carry fear, uncertainty, past experiences, financial concerns, and often the silent pressure of their family's expectations.

All of this converges at one point: the doctor.

In moments of illness, especially when the condition is serious or unclear, the mind naturally seeks stability. Patients and their families look for someone who appears confident, composed, and capable of handling the situation.

The doctor becomes that anchor.

This process is not always conscious. It is a psychological response. When uncertainty increases, the need for assurance also increases. The doctor, by virtue of their role, becomes the focal point for this need.

Expectations begin to build—not just from logic, but from emotion.

Patients may expect immediate clarity: *What exactly is the problem? How serious is it? What will happen next?* Families often expect a timeline: *When will recovery begin? How long will it take? Will everything return to normal?*

These questions are natural.

But medicine does not always provide immediate or definitive answers. Diagnosis can take time. Conditions can evolve. Treatments may require adjustment. Outcomes may vary depending on multiple factors.

Yet the emotional need for certainty remains urgent.

This creates a gap between what patients need emotionally and what medicine can offer realistically. To bridge this gap, patients often project their expectations onto the doctor. They assume that the doctor must have answers—even when the situation itself is still unfolding.

The doctor becomes the carrier of certainty.

Families, especially in collective cultures, add another layer to this dynamic. Multiple members may be involved in decision-making, each bringing their own concerns, opinions, and expectations. The doctor must address not just one individual, but an entire emotional system.

The interaction becomes multi-directional.

In critical situations, this projection intensifies. When outcomes are uncertain or unfavorable, the emotional weight increases. Families may seek reassurance repeatedly, ask for guarantees, or expect constant availability and updates.

The doctor becomes the center of emotional gravity.

What is often overlooked is that this emotional projection is not about mistrust—it is about dependence. In moments of vulnerability, people naturally depend on someone who appears to have control over the situation.

The doctor represents that control.

However, this dependence can place significant pressure on the doctor. They must manage not only the medical condition but also the emotional expectations surrounding it. They must communicate carefully—providing information without creating false assurance, showing empathy without promising certainty.

This requires balance.

Too much clinical detachment may appear insensitive. Too much reassurance may create unrealistic expectations. The doctor must navigate this space continuously, often within limited time and under significant pressure.

The emotional landscape becomes part of the consultation.

Understanding this dynamic is important for both sides. Patients and families need to recognize that their emotional responses are natural, but the doctor cannot always fulfill the need for certainty. Doctors, in turn, must acknowledge the emotional reality of patients and respond with clarity and empathy.

Because healing is not only biological—it is also psychological.

And in that psychological space, the doctor is not just treating a condition.

They are managing the weight of expectations that arise when human vulnerability meets the search for stability.

11.5 — The Impact of Unrealistic Expectations on Doctors

When expectations quietly exceed the limits of medicine, the pressure does not disappear—it transfers. And it is the doctor who absorbs it.

In modern practice, doctors are not only required to make correct decisions; they are expected to make perfect decisions.

Every diagnosis must be accurate, every treatment must work, every outcome must align with expectation. The tolerance for error, delay, or uncertainty has narrowed significantly, even though the complexity of cases has increased.

This creates a constant background pressure.

Doctors begin to operate in an environment where the cost of a mistake—real or perceived—is extremely high. A missed diagnosis can lead to legal consequences. A complication, even if unavoidable, may be interpreted as negligence. A delay in recovery may be seen as failure.

The margin for human limitation becomes smaller.

This pressure directly affects decision-making.

In some situations, doctors may adopt defensive approaches—ordering additional tests not only for clinical clarity but also to reduce risk. They may become cautious in communication, choosing words carefully to avoid misinterpretation. Decisions are influenced not only by medical reasoning but also by the potential consequences of how those decisions will be perceived.

Clinical judgment begins to carry an additional layer of calculation.

Over time, this environment contributes to mental fatigue.

Doctors are required to remain alert, responsible, and composed across long hours and multiple patients. When unrealistic expectations are added to this workload, the cognitive load increases further. Each case is not only a medical challenge but also a potential point of scrutiny.

The mind rarely gets rest.

Emotionally, the impact can be even deeper.

Doctors are trained to maintain composure, but they are not unaffected by outcomes. When a patient does not improve, or when complications arise, doctors carry that experience with them. When, in addition to this, they face dissatisfaction or blame despite sincere effort, the emotional burden increases.

Effort and outcome begin to feel disconnected.

This can lead to a gradual shift in behavior.

Some doctors may become more detached as a way to protect themselves. Others may limit communication to avoid extended discussions that could lead to conflict. In certain cases, enthusiasm for the profession may reduce, replaced by a more mechanical approach to work.

The profession begins to lose its internal motivation.

Burnout becomes a real risk.

Long hours, high responsibility, and constant pressure without adequate emotional support can lead to exhaustion—both physical and psychological. Burnout does not always appear dramatically; it often develops slowly, reflected in reduced engagement, irritability, or a sense of detachment from work.

The system continues, but the individual begins to withdraw.

At a broader level, unrealistic expectations also affect the doctor–patient relationship.

When expectations are not met, even if the doctor has acted appropriately, dissatisfaction can arise. This can lead to conflict, mistrust, or strained communication. Doctors may begin to anticipate these reactions, which further influences how they interact with patients.

The relationship becomes guarded.

Understanding this impact is essential.

Doctors are not resistant to responsibility—they have chosen a profession that inherently carries it. What becomes difficult is when responsibility is combined with expectations that do not align with the nature of medicine itself.

Because medicine operates within uncertainty.

Recognizing the limits of what doctors can control does not reduce their importance—it makes their role more realistic. It allows space for effort to be acknowledged, even when outcomes vary.

And it allows doctors to function not as flawless performers, but as skilled professionals working within a complex and unpredictable system.

11.6 — When Expectations Turn into Conflict

When expectations remain aligned with reality, the doctor–patient relationship functions as a collaborative process. There is trust, communication, and a shared effort toward recovery.

But when expectations exceed what medicine can deliver, that alignment begins to break.

And when alignment breaks, tension enters the interaction.

Conflict in healthcare rarely begins with hostility. It usually begins with a gap—between what the patient or family expected and what actually happens. A diagnosis takes longer than anticipated. A treatment does not produce immediate results. Recovery is slower, incomplete, or uncertain.

The expectation was certainty. The reality is complexity.

In that moment, dissatisfaction begins to form.

Patients and families, already under emotional stress, may interpret the gap as a failure of the doctor rather than a limitation of the situation. Questions become sharper. Doubts begin to surface. The tone of communication shifts—from seeking understanding to seeking justification.

The conversation becomes defensive on both sides.

Doctors, sensing this shift, may respond by becoming more cautious in their communication. They may limit explanations, avoid extended discussions, or rely strictly on clinical language to reduce ambiguity. While this approach may protect against misinterpretation, it can also reduce the sense of connection.

The interaction loses warmth.

This creates a feedback loop.

Reduced communication from the doctor increases uncertainty for the patient. Increased uncertainty intensifies emotional reactions. Stronger emotional reactions further strain communication. The cycle continues, often escalating without either side intending it.

Misunderstanding grows silently.

In some cases, this escalation can lead to open conflict.

Arguments may arise over treatment decisions, perceived delays, or outcomes. Families may demand explanations or accountability in ways that reflect their frustration and fear. Doctors may feel that their professional judgment is being questioned despite sincere effort.

The relationship shifts from trust to confrontation.

Legal awareness also plays a role in this dynamic.

In environments where medical decisions are subject to scrutiny, both doctors and patients become more guarded. Patients may approach interactions with a sense of caution, while doctors may practice defensively to protect themselves from potential allegations.

The system becomes more formal, but less human.

In extreme situations, conflicts can extend beyond communication into serious disputes. These are not always a result of negligence; they often arise from accumulated frustration, emotional stress, and unmet expectations.

The underlying issue remains the same: misalignment.

What makes this particularly challenging is that both sides are, in their own way, justified. Patients seek clarity, assurance, and the best possible outcome. Doctors aim to apply their knowledge responsibly within the limits of medicine.

But when expectations are not aligned with those limits, even appropriate care can be perceived as inadequate.

Resolving this requires more than better systems or stricter rules. It requires recognition.

Patients and families need to understand that medicine does not operate with guarantees. Doctors need to acknowledge the emotional intensity that patients experience and communicate with clarity and empathy.

Alignment must be rebuilt consciously.

Because conflict in healthcare is rarely about opposition—it is about expectation exceeding reality.

And when that gap is understood and addressed, the relationship can move back from confrontation to collaboration, where both sides work together toward the same goal: recovery and well-being.

11.7 — Reframing Expectations: A Shared Responsibility

If unrealistic expectations are the source of strain, then the solution does not lie in reducing expectations alone—it lies in reframing them.

Reframing does not weaken the role of the doctor. It strengthens the understanding of the system.

At the center of this shift is a simple realization: healthcare is not a one-sided service—it is a participatory process. The outcome of treatment is influenced not only by the doctor's knowledge but also by the patient's condition, response to treatment, timing, and adherence to advice.

Responsibility is distributed, not isolated.

For society, this means moving away from the idea of the doctor as a miracle worker. Doctors are highly trained professionals, but they operate within biological uncertainty. Not every disease can be cured, not every condition can be reversed, and not every outcome can be controlled.

Accepting this does not reduce trust—it makes it more realistic.

Patients and families play a crucial role in this reframing.

They must engage with the process actively—by sharing accurate information, following treatment plans, asking questions with the intent to understand, and recognizing that recovery may take time. Trust must be accompanied by participation.

Care becomes a shared effort.

At the same time, doctors must also adapt.

Clear and transparent communication becomes essential. Explaining not only the diagnosis but also the uncertainties, possible outcomes, and limitations of treatment helps align expectations early. When patients understand the range of possibilities, they are better prepared for the journey ahead.

Clarity reduces conflict.

Empathy remains equally important.

Patients do not approach healthcare as neutral participants—they come with fear and vulnerability. Recognizing this emotional context and responding with patience and understanding helps build trust, even when outcomes are uncertain.

Connection supports cooperation.

Healthcare institutions also have a role to play.

Systems must allow adequate time for doctor–patient interaction, support clear communication, and reduce unnecessary administrative burdens that limit meaningful engagement. When systems prioritize efficiency alone, the human aspect of care is often compromised.

Structure influences behavior.

At a broader level, public awareness becomes critical.

Society must develop a more accurate understanding of what medicine can and cannot do. This includes acknowledging uncertainty, variability in outcomes, and the complexity of biological systems. Education—formal or informal—can help bridge the gap between perception and reality.

Awareness creates alignment.

Regulatory frameworks and policies must also support this balance.

They should protect patient rights while also recognizing the challenges doctors face. Systems that are overly punitive can create fear, while systems that lack accountability can reduce trust. The goal is to maintain equilibrium.

Balance sustains the system.

Ultimately, reframing expectations is about restoring a partnership.

The doctor is not the sole bearer of responsibility, and the patient is not a passive recipient of care. Both are participants in a process that aims to achieve the best possible outcome within the limits of medicine.

When this partnership is understood, the burden becomes shared.

And when the burden is shared, the relationship becomes stronger.

Because healthcare functions best not when one side expects everything from the other, but when both sides align with the reality of the system and work together within it.

The Human Behind the White Coat

At the heart of all expectations, systems, and structures, there remains a simple truth that is often overlooked:

The doctor is human.

Behind the white coat is not an infallible authority, but an individual who has studied deeply, trained rigorously, and chosen a profession that places them at the intersection of knowledge, responsibility, and uncertainty. They think, they decide, they carry outcomes—and they are affected by them.

Yet the role they occupy often hides this reality.

Patients see confidence, not the internal calculation behind decisions. They see authority, not the years of doubt, correction, and learning that shaped that authority. They see answers, not the uncertainty that often exists behind those answers.

The human layer becomes invisible.

This invisibility is reinforced by the expectations placed on the profession. Doctors are expected to remain composed in crisis, clear in uncertainty, and stable under pressure. They are expected to deliver difficult information with sensitivity, manage complex situations with precision, and continue functioning regardless of emotional strain.

They are expected to absorb without showing.

But no professional, regardless of training, is beyond human limitation.

Doctors experience fatigue, especially in systems that demand long hours and constant attention. They experience emotional impact when outcomes are not favorable. They carry the weight of decisions that affect lives, sometimes long after the consultation has ended.

The responsibility does not end with the interaction.

Recognizing the human behind the white coat does not reduce the expectation of competence—it contextualizes it. It allows society to maintain trust while also acknowledging that medicine operates through individuals who function within limits.

This recognition changes the nature of interaction.

When patients see doctors not as distant authorities but as skilled professionals working within complexity, communication becomes more open. Questions become collaborative rather than confrontational. Outcomes, whether positive or negative, are understood within a broader context.

The relationship becomes more balanced.

For doctors, this recognition also matters.

It allows them to practice with awareness rather than fear, to communicate honestly without the pressure of unrealistic perfection, and to engage with patients as participants rather than performers.

It restores authenticity to the profession.

The white coat, then, should not be seen as a shield that hides human reality, nor as a symbol that demands perfection. It should be understood as a responsibility carried by a human being—one who applies knowledge, judgment, and effort in situations where certainty is not always possible.

That understanding does not weaken trust.

It strengthens it.

Because trust built on unrealistic expectations is fragile. Trust built on understanding is resilient.

And in a profession where every interaction carries weight, resilience is what sustains both the doctor and the patient through the realities of healthcare.

Reflective Interlude

Between Expectation and Reality

Somewhere between the system and the individual, between science and society, a quiet distortion has taken place.

Not dramatic. Not sudden. But deep enough to change how medicine is experienced.

Doctors feel burdened. Patients feel dissatisfied. And both believe the other side has changed.

But the truth is simpler.

The system has expanded faster than understanding.

Medicine has advanced, but expectations have grown even faster. Institutions have scaled, but human connection has thinned. Information has increased, but clarity has not kept pace.

We are standing in a system that works—but does not always feel right.

The doctor today is not the same as the doctor of the past. Not because the intention has changed, but because the environment has.

More patients.

Less time.

More accountability.

Less margin for error.

More information.

Less trust.

The role has stretched.

At the same time, the patient is not the same as before.

More aware.

More anxious.

More demanding.

Less patient.

More informed—but not always aligned.

The interaction has changed.

And in between these two evolving realities, something essential has been lost—not completely, but enough to be noticed.

Clarity of role.

The doctor is trying to function within systems. The patient is trying to find certainty within uncertainty. Both are right in their own space.

But the alignment is missing.

This misalignment is not a failure of individuals. It is a result of a system that has grown without redefining its core relationships.

We have improved medicine. But we have not redefined what it means to be a doctor in this new world.

That is the gap we now face.

Because continuing with old expectations in a new system will only increase friction. And reducing expectations without redefining purpose will only reduce trust.

What is required is something else.

A redefinition.

Not of medicine. But of the doctor's role within it.

A shift from image to function. From expectation to alignment. From assumption to understanding.

Because if the system has changed, then the role within the system must also be understood again.

And that is where we move next.

Not to criticize what exists. But to redefine what it should mean—today—to be a doctor.

PART IV — REDEFINING THE DOCTOR

A doctor is not defined by knowledge alone, but by how that knowledge is carried in the presence of another human being.

Chapter 12 — Clinical Skill and Human Intelligence

Beyond Knowledge

There was a time when knowledge itself was the defining strength of a doctor.

The ability to recall symptoms, identify diseases, and prescribe treatment distinguished a physician from the rest of society. Information was scarce, access was limited, and medical knowledge carried both authority and power.

But that landscape has changed.

Today, information is everywhere. Patients arrive with reports, online research, second opinions, and pre-formed questions. Medical knowledge, at least in its basic form, is no longer exclusive to the doctor. The gap between what the doctor knows and what the patient can access has narrowed.

Yet something crucial remains unchanged.

The ability to *decide*.

Medicine has never been just about knowing. It has always been about interpreting, prioritizing, and acting under uncertainty. Two doctors can possess the same knowledge, read the same reports, and still arrive at different conclusions.

Because knowledge does not make decisions. Intelligence does.

In real clinical settings, information rarely presents itself in complete form. Symptoms are vague, histories are incomplete, and conditions evolve over time. The doctor must filter noise, identify patterns, and choose a path forward—often without the luxury of certainty.

This is where knowledge reaches its limit.

A textbook can describe a disease, but it cannot capture every variation of how it appears in real life. Guidelines can suggest protocols, but they cannot account for every individual difference. Reports can provide data, but they do not interpret themselves.

The doctor must bridge the gap.

This bridge is built not only on knowledge, but on clinical skill and human intelligence—the ability to observe carefully, think critically, adapt to changing conditions, and respond with clarity.

It is the difference between information and understanding.

Patients may not always recognize the depth of knowledge a doctor possesses, but they immediately sense the quality of decisions. They notice whether the doctor listens, whether the explanation makes sense, whether the approach feels thoughtful and aligned with their condition.

Trust is formed in these moments.

In modern medicine, therefore, the defining factor is no longer how much a doctor knows, but how effectively they use what they know. Knowledge is the foundation, but intelligence determines its application.

And application determines outcome.

This shift is subtle but significant.

It requires doctors to move beyond accumulation toward integration. It requires them to think, not just recall. It requires them to engage with each case as a dynamic situation rather than a predefined problem.

Because in the end, medicine is not practiced in textbooks.

It is practiced in real time, with real people, where decisions matter more than information—and where intelligence transforms knowledge into care.

12.1 — The Limits of Medical Knowledge

Medical knowledge is vast, structured, and continuously expanding. Textbooks, research papers, clinical guidelines, and protocols provide a comprehensive framework for understanding diseases, their causes, and their treatment. This body of knowledge forms the foundation of modern medicine.

But a foundation, by itself, does not complete the structure.

One of the fundamental realities of medicine is that it operates within probabilities, not certainties. A disease may have a typical presentation, but not every patient will follow that pattern. A treatment may be effective in most cases, but not in all. Outcomes are influenced by multiple variables—genetics, environment, timing, co-existing conditions, and individual response.

Knowledge defines possibilities. Reality presents variations.

Textbooks are designed to simplify complexity. They describe conditions in organized formats—symptoms, causes, investigations, and treatments. This structure is essential for learning, but it creates an implicit assumption that diseases behave in predictable ways.

In practice, they often do not.

A patient may present with incomplete or misleading symptoms. Early stages of disease may not show clear signs. Multiple conditions may overlap, creating confusion. In such situations, the doctor must work with partial information.

Knowledge alone cannot resolve uncertainty.

Clinical guidelines attempt to standardize care by providing recommended pathways for diagnosis and treatment. They are based on large-scale data and evidence, offering valuable direction. However, these guidelines are designed for general populations, not for every individual case.

Every patient introduces exceptions.

Strictly following protocols without considering context can lead to inappropriate decisions. A treatment suitable for one patient may not be ideal for another due to differences in age, medical history, or overall condition.

This is where the limitation of knowledge becomes visible.

Another aspect of this limitation is the dynamic nature of medicine itself. New research continuously updates understanding. Treatments that were considered standard in the past may be replaced by more effective approaches. What is known today may evolve tomorrow.

Knowledge is not static.

Doctors must therefore operate with an awareness that their knowledge, while essential, is always incomplete in some sense. This does not weaken the profession—it defines its nature. Medicine is a field where learning continues, and certainty is rarely absolute.

This requires humility.

Patients, however, often expect definitive answers. They assume that medical knowledge is complete and that every condition has a clear explanation and solution. When doctors express uncertainty or require time for diagnosis, it may be perceived as a lack of competence.

But in reality, it reflects the complexity of the field.

Understanding the limits of medical knowledge is crucial for both doctors and patients. For doctors, it reinforces the need to go beyond information and develop judgment. For patients, it helps align expectations with the realities of medical practice.

Because knowledge, no matter how extensive, cannot cover every scenario.

It must be interpreted, adapted, and applied—within the limits of what is known and the uncertainties that remain.

12.2 — Clinical Skill: The Art of Application

If knowledge defines what is possible, clinical skill determines what is done.

It is the bridge between theory and reality.

A doctor may understand diseases in depth, recall protocols accurately, and interpret investigations correctly in isolation. But in practice, these elements do not arrive in sequence or in perfect clarity. They appear together—often incomplete, sometimes conflicting, and always time-sensitive.

Clinical skill is the ability to navigate this complexity.

It begins with observation.

A skilled clinician does not merely look at reports; they observe the patient. Posture, tone of voice, breathing pattern, facial expression—these subtle cues often carry information that no test can capture. A patient's history is not just a list of symptoms; it is a narrative that requires careful listening and interpretation.

What is said matters. What is not said matters equally.

From observation, the doctor moves to pattern recognition.

Over time, exposure to multiple cases allows doctors to identify recurring patterns—combinations of symptoms, timelines, and responses that suggest particular conditions. This recognition is not mechanical; it is intuitive, built through experience and reflection.

It allows the doctor to move from possibility to probability.

But patterns are not always clear.

In many cases, information is incomplete or ambiguous. Symptoms may overlap across multiple conditions. Investigations may not provide definitive answers. The doctor must then make decisions based on partial data, weighing risks and benefits while considering the patient's overall context.

This is where judgment becomes critical.

Clinical skill involves prioritization.

Not every symptom requires equal attention. Not every test is necessary. Not every treatment should be initiated immediately. The doctor must decide what matters most at a given moment—what to address first, what to monitor, and what to defer.

This prioritization shapes outcomes.

Time is another dimension of clinical skill.

Decisions often need to be made quickly, especially in acute settings. There is limited opportunity for extended analysis. The doctor must act with confidence while remaining open to revising the decision as new information emerges.

Action and adaptability must coexist.

Experience plays a central role in developing this ability.

Repeated exposure to real cases refines judgment. Mistakes, reflections, and corrections contribute to deeper understanding. Over time, the doctor develops an internal framework—a way of thinking that integrates knowledge, observation, and experience into a coherent approach.

This framework cannot be memorized. It must be built.

Clinical skill also includes knowing when not to act.

Restraint is as important as intervention. Unnecessary tests, premature treatments, or overreaction to uncertain findings can create complications. A skilled doctor understands when observation is more appropriate than immediate action.

Doing less can sometimes achieve more.

Communication is embedded within clinical skill.

Explaining decisions, discussing uncertainties, and guiding patients through the process require clarity and confidence. A decision, no matter how correct, loses value if it is not understood by the patient.

Understanding strengthens trust.

Ultimately, clinical skill transforms knowledge into meaningful action. It is not visible in certificates or degrees, but it becomes evident in how a doctor approaches each case, adapts to challenges, and makes decisions under pressure.

It is the difference between knowing medicine and practicing it.

And in a field where every decision carries consequence, that difference defines the quality of care.

12.3 — Human Intelligence in Medicine

When we speak about intelligence in medicine, it is often assumed to mean academic ability—the capacity to understand complex concepts, remember large volumes of information, and perform well in examinations.

But real medical practice demands a broader form of intelligence.

It is not limited to what the doctor knows. It is defined by how the doctor perceives, adapts, and responds.

Human intelligence in medicine begins with awareness.

A doctor must be aware not only of the disease but also of the context in which it exists. A patient's condition is influenced by their lifestyle, emotional state, family environment, and even their ability to follow treatment. Recognizing these factors requires attention beyond clinical data.

The situation must be understood, not just the symptom.

This awareness extends to the clinical environment itself.

A patient's condition can change rapidly. New information may emerge. Investigations may reveal unexpected findings. A doctor must remain alert to these shifts and adjust their approach accordingly.

Static thinking does not work in a dynamic system.

Adaptability, therefore, becomes a key component of intelligence.

Medical situations rarely follow a fixed path. A treatment that works for one patient may not work for another. A diagnosis may need revision as new evidence appears. Doctors must be willing to update their understanding and modify their decisions without hesitation.

Flexibility supports accuracy.

Emotional intelligence is equally important.

Patients are not neutral participants; they come with fear, anxiety, and expectations. A doctor must be able to recognize these emotional states and respond appropriately. This does not mean becoming emotionally involved in every case, but it requires sensitivity to how patients experience their condition.

Communication depends on this sensitivity.

A patient who feels heard is more likely to trust the process. A family that understands the situation is less likely to react with frustration. Emotional intelligence, therefore, directly influences the effectiveness of medical care.

It shapes the interaction.

Another dimension of human intelligence is judgment under uncertainty.

In many situations, there is no single correct answer. The doctor must evaluate multiple possibilities, consider risks, and choose a course of action. This requires the ability to think clearly even when information is incomplete.

Clarity must exist within uncertainty.

This form of intelligence also includes self-awareness.

Doctors must recognize the limits of their knowledge, the possibility of error, and the need for consultation when required. Confidence is necessary, but overconfidence can be dangerous. Balancing these aspects requires continuous reflection.

Awareness of self improves decisions.

Human intelligence in medicine is not developed through textbooks alone.

It grows through experience, observation, interaction, and reflection. It evolves with each patient, each case, and each outcome. Over time, it becomes an internal system that guides how a doctor thinks and acts.

It is shaped by practice.

In modern healthcare, where information is abundant and systems are complex, this form of intelligence becomes even more critical. Knowledge can be accessed, protocols can be followed, but the ability to interpret and apply them effectively depends on human intelligence.

And that cannot be standardized.

Ultimately, human intelligence is what allows a doctor to function not just as a technical expert, but as a responsive and adaptive professional—one who can navigate complexity while maintaining clarity.

Because medicine is not practiced in controlled conditions.

It is practiced in real life, where variables change, people differ, and decisions must be made with both knowledge and understanding working together.

12.4 — The Doctor as a Thinking System

In modern medicine, a doctor is not simply applying knowledge—they are continuously processing information, filtering variables, and making decisions in real time.

In many ways, the doctor functions as a *thinking system*.

Every patient interaction brings multiple layers of input. There is the biological layer—symptoms, signs, investigations, medical history. But alongside this, there is a psychological layer—fear, anxiety, expectations. There is also a social layer—family dynamics, financial constraints, lifestyle factors.

All of these arrive together.

The doctor must integrate them into a coherent understanding. A symptom is not interpreted in isolation; it is evaluated in relation to other findings. A test result is not taken at face value; it is considered in the context of the patient's overall condition.

Meaning emerges through integration.

This integration requires continuous filtering.

Not all information is equally important. Some details are critical, others are noise. A doctor must quickly identify what matters, what can be temporarily set aside, and what requires immediate attention.

This is prioritization in action.

At the same time, the doctor is constantly evaluating risk.

Every decision carries consequences. Ordering a test has implications—cost, time, and possible findings. Starting a treatment involves potential benefits and side effects. Delaying action may allow more clarity but also carries risk.

The doctor must balance these factors.

This balance is rarely straightforward. There is often no option that is entirely safe or entirely certain. The doctor must choose the most appropriate path based on available information, understanding that outcomes cannot be guaranteed.

Decision-making becomes a calculated judgment.

Time adds another dimension.

In many situations, especially emergencies, decisions must be made quickly. There is limited opportunity for extended analysis. The doctor must rely on their internal framework—built through knowledge and experience—to act efficiently.

Speed and accuracy must coexist.

The thinking system is also dynamic.

As new information becomes available—new symptoms, updated reports, patient response—the doctor must revise their understanding. A diagnosis may be refined, a treatment plan may be adjusted, and the course of action may change.

Flexibility is built into the system.

This continuous loop—observe, interpret, decide, act, reassess—defines clinical practice.

It is not a linear process. It is iterative, adaptive, and responsive to change. The doctor is constantly updating their internal model of the patient's condition.

Thinking is ongoing, not episodic.

What makes this system particularly complex is that it operates under pressure.

Time constraints, patient expectations, institutional demands, and the inherent uncertainty of medicine all influence how decisions are made. Despite these pressures, the doctor is expected to maintain clarity and consistency.

The system must remain stable under load.

This is why the role of the doctor cannot be reduced to protocols or algorithms alone.

Guidelines can support decision-making, but they cannot replace the integration of multiple variables in real time. The doctor's thinking system is what allows adaptation when situations deviate from standard patterns.

It enables responsiveness.

Understanding the doctor as a thinking system helps shift the focus from isolated knowledge to integrated intelligence. It highlights that the value of a doctor lies not only in what they know, but in how they process, connect, and act on that knowledge.

Because in the end, medicine is not a set of instructions.

It is a continuous process of thinking—where each decision is shaped by multiple inputs, evolving conditions, and the responsibility to choose the best possible path forward.

12.5 — When Knowledge Without Intelligence Fails

In theory, medicine appears structured and predictable. There are established protocols, standardized guidelines, and well-documented treatment pathways. A doctor who knows these thoroughly should, in principle, be able to manage most situations effectively.

But practice tells a different story.

There are moments when everything appears correct on paper—tests ordered appropriately, protocols followed, medications prescribed as per guidelines—yet the outcome is not as expected. The condition does not improve, complications arise, or the patient's situation worsens.

The knowledge was correct. The outcome was not.

This gap reveals an important truth: knowledge, when applied without intelligence, can fail.

One common example is the over-reliance on protocols.

Guidelines are designed to assist decision-making, but they are based on generalized data. When applied rigidly, without considering the unique context of a patient, they can lead to decisions that are technically correct but practically inappropriate.

The system was followed, but the situation was not understood.

Another failure occurs when clinical context is ignored.

A patient is not just a collection of symptoms. They have a history, lifestyle, emotional state, and social environment that influence both the disease and the treatment. Applying knowledge without considering these factors reduces medicine to a mechanical process.

The human dimension is lost.

In some cases, excessive dependence on investigations replaces clinical judgment.

Doctors may rely heavily on reports and imaging, expecting definitive answers. While these tools are valuable, they do not interpret themselves. Without proper clinical correlation, they can mislead or create unnecessary complexity.

Data without interpretation becomes noise.

Timing also plays a critical role.

Knowing what to do is different from knowing *when* to do it. A treatment given too early, too late, or without proper assessment can alter outcomes significantly. Clinical intelligence involves understanding the sequence and timing of actions.

Right action at the wrong time is still a wrong decision.

Communication failures can also arise from knowledge without intelligence.

A doctor may understand the condition perfectly but fail to explain it in a way the patient can understand. This can lead to confusion, lack of compliance, or mistrust. In such cases, the problem is not medical—it is interpretational.

Understanding must be shared, not just possessed.

There is also the risk of overconfidence.

A doctor who relies solely on knowledge may assume certainty where none exists. This can lead to premature conclusions, overlooking alternative possibilities, or resisting reassessment when new information emerges.

Intelligence requires openness.

In contrast, clinical intelligence introduces flexibility.

It allows the doctor to question, to adapt, to reconsider, and to integrate multiple dimensions of a case. It recognizes that knowledge provides a framework, but real situations require interpretation beyond that framework.

It balances structure with awareness.

Patients often sense this difference, even if they cannot articulate it. They recognize when a doctor is simply following a process versus when a doctor is truly engaging with their situation. The latter builds confidence; the former may feel impersonal or incomplete.

Trust is influenced by perception of thinking.

Understanding when knowledge fails is not a criticism of learning—it is a reminder of its limits. It highlights the need to move beyond accumulation toward application, beyond correctness toward appropriateness.

Because in medicine, the goal is not to apply knowledge perfectly.

It is to apply it intelligently—within the context of a real human situation, where variables are many and certainty is rare.

12.6 — Building Intelligence Alongside Knowledge

If knowledge forms the base of medicine, then intelligence must be cultivated deliberately as its operating system. It does not emerge automatically from studying textbooks or passing examinations. It develops through structured exposure, guided thinking, and continuous reflection.

The first shift required is in how learning itself is approached.

Medical education must move beyond information delivery toward problem engagement. Instead of asking *"What is this disease?"*, students must be trained to ask *"What is happening in this patient?"* This shift transforms learning from static recall to dynamic interpretation.

Learning becomes situational.

Case-based learning is one of the most effective tools in this process.

Real or simulated cases expose students to the complexity of clinical scenarios. They must interpret symptoms, evaluate possibilities, prioritize actions, and justify decisions. This method forces integration of knowledge rather than isolated recall.

Cases teach thinking.

Equally important is reflective practice.

After every clinical interaction—successful or otherwise—there must be space to reflect. What was observed? What decision was made? What could have been done differently? Reflection converts experience into insight.

Without reflection, experience remains incomplete.

Mentorship plays a critical role in shaping intelligence.

Experienced clinicians do more than demonstrate outcomes; they reveal their thinking. They explain why a particular decision was made, what alternatives were considered, and how uncertainty was handled. Observing this process allows students to internalize patterns of reasoning.

Thinking is transferred through interaction.

Exposure to variability is also essential.

Students must encounter a wide range of cases—common conditions, rare presentations, straightforward diagnoses, and ambiguous situations. This diversity builds adaptability and prevents rigid thinking.

Variation strengthens flexibility.

Simulation and controlled environments can support early development.

Simulated cases, skill labs, and scenario-based training allow students to practice decision-making without immediate risk to patients. These environments provide opportunities to make mistakes, learn from them, and refine judgment.

Practice builds confidence.

However, no simulation can replace real patient interaction.

Direct engagement with patients introduces unpredictability, emotional context, and the responsibility of real outcomes. This experience anchors intelligence in reality and reinforces the importance of careful decision-making.

Reality shapes maturity.

Continuous learning must extend beyond formal education.

Medicine evolves, and so must the doctor's thinking. Attending discussions, reviewing cases, engaging with new research, and learning from peers all contribute to ongoing development. Intelligence is not fixed—it grows with exposure and effort.

Learning never ends.

Self-awareness is another key component.

Doctors must recognize their strengths and limitations. Knowing when to seek a second opinion, when to reconsider a decision, or when to pause and reassess is part of intelligent practice.

Awareness protects against error.

Institutional culture also influences this process.

Environments that encourage questioning, discussion, and learning from mistakes foster deeper intelligence. In contrast, systems that prioritize only performance or discourage inquiry may limit the development of critical thinking.

Culture shapes cognition.

Ultimately, building intelligence alongside knowledge requires intentional design—at the level of education, mentorship, and practice. It is not an additional skill but an integral part of becoming a competent doctor.

Because knowledge provides the tools.

But intelligence determines how, when, and why those tools are used—and in medicine, that distinction defines the quality of care.

12.7 — Trust Is Built on Decisions, Not Degrees

A medical degree establishes entry into the profession. It signals that a doctor has undergone formal training, met academic requirements, and is qualified to practice.

But for a patient, trust does not begin with the degree.

It begins with the decision.

Patients rarely evaluate a doctor based on where they studied or how many distinctions they achieved. These details may carry initial weight, but they fade quickly in the face of real interaction. What remains is the experience—how the doctor listens, how they interpret the situation, and how they guide the patient forward.

Trust forms in real time.

A patient observes whether the doctor pays attention to their concerns or moves quickly through the consultation. They notice whether the explanation is clear or confusing. They sense whether the approach is thoughtful or mechanical.

These observations shape confidence.

The quality of decisions plays a central role in this process.

A well-considered diagnosis, a logical treatment plan, and an explanation that connects all elements together create a sense of alignment. Even when outcomes are uncertain, patients feel reassured when they understand the reasoning behind the decisions.

Clarity builds trust.

Consistency strengthens it further.

When a doctor demonstrates stable judgment across multiple interactions—when their approach remains logical, adaptable, and patient-centered—confidence deepens. Patients begin to rely not just on individual decisions but on the pattern of thinking behind them.

Trust becomes cumulative.

On the other hand, when decisions appear inconsistent, unclear, or disconnected from the patient's experience, doubt begins to emerge. Even if the underlying knowledge is sound, the lack of visible reasoning can create uncertainty.

Trust weakens when thinking is not visible.

Communication becomes the bridge.

A decision that is not explained remains incomplete from the patient's perspective. Patients need to understand not only what is being done but why it is being done. When doctors articulate their reasoning, they allow patients to participate in the process.

Understanding transforms compliance into cooperation.

This is particularly important in complex or long-term conditions.

Patients must often follow treatment plans over extended periods, adapt to changes, and make decisions about their own care. When they trust the doctor's thinking, they are more likely to remain engaged and committed to the process.

Trust supports continuity.

It is also important to recognize that trust is resilient when built on understanding.

If outcomes are not as expected, patients who trust the doctor's judgment are more likely to accept the situation as part of the uncertainty of medicine. They differentiate between effort and outcome, recognizing that not all variables are controllable.

Trust absorbs uncertainty.

This does not mean that degrees and qualifications are irrelevant.

They provide the foundation that allows doctors to practice. But they are not sufficient to sustain trust. Trust must be earned repeatedly through decisions, interactions, and communication.

It is built, not assumed.

In modern medicine, where information is accessible and expectations are high, patients are not only looking for knowledge—they are looking for clarity, reasoning, and reliability.

They are looking for intelligence in action.

Because at the moment of decision, when a patient places their health in a doctor's hands, what matters most is not the certificate on the wall.

It is the confidence that the decision being made is thoughtful, appropriate, and aligned with their situation.

The Intelligent Doctor

In the end, the evolution of medicine is not only about better drugs, advanced machines, or improved protocols.

It is about better thinking.

A doctor may carry extensive knowledge, possess advanced tools, and operate within a sophisticated system. But when a patient sits in front of them, all of that condenses into a single moment—the moment of decision.

And in that moment, what matters is not how much is known, but how well it is used.

The intelligent doctor is not defined by perfection.

They are defined by awareness.

Awareness of what is known and what is not. Awareness of the patient as a person, not just a condition. Awareness of the risks, limitations, and consequences of each decision.

This awareness creates balance.

The intelligent doctor does not rush to conclusions, nor do they hesitate unnecessarily. They move with clarity, but without arrogance. They are confident, but open to revision. They act, but remain ready to adapt.

Their strength lies in alignment, not certainty.

In a world where information is abundant, the value of intelligence becomes even more visible. Patients may arrive informed, systems may provide data, and technology may assist in diagnosis—but the responsibility to interpret and act still rests with the doctor.

The human element cannot be replaced.

This is where the future of trust in medicine will be decided.

Not by the accumulation of knowledge alone, but by the quality of decisions made in complex, uncertain situations. Patients will continue to seek doctors who not only know but understand, who not only diagnose but think, who not only treat but guide.

They will seek intelligence in action.

For doctors, this redefinition carries both challenge and opportunity.

The challenge is to move beyond traditional measures of competence and develop deeper cognitive and perceptual abilities. The opportunity is to reclaim the essence of the profession—not as a repository of knowledge, but as a living application of it.

A profession grounded in thinking.

The intelligent doctor does not separate science from humanity. They integrate both. They recognize that medicine is not just about correcting biological processes, but about engaging with human life in all its complexity.

They treat with understanding.

And perhaps most importantly, they remain learners.

They observe, reflect, adapt, and evolve. Each patient becomes a source of insight. Each decision becomes part of a growing framework of understanding. Intelligence is not a fixed state—it is a continuous process.

It grows with practice.

As medicine continues to advance, this distinction will only become more important. Knowledge will expand, systems will become more complex, and expectations will continue to rise.

But the core will remain the same.

A doctor, standing at the intersection of knowledge and uncertainty, making decisions that matter.

And in that space, the difference between a good doctor and a truly trusted one will not be defined by what they know.

It will be defined by how intelligently they think.

Chapter 13 — The Responsibility of Authority

The Weight of a Decision

There are moments in medicine that pass quietly, without announcement, yet carry the power to change a life completely.

A diagnosis is confirmed. A treatment is initiated. A surgery is approved. A decision is made.

From the outside, it may appear routine. Part of the process. Another step in a system that runs every day, across hospitals and clinics, across cities and countries.

But for the patient, that moment is not routine.

It is decisive.

A single decision can determine the direction of recovery, the possibility of complications, the length of suffering, or, in some cases, the boundary between life and death. It can influence not only the patient's condition but also the lives of their family, their work, their future.

The impact extends far beyond the consultation room.

For the doctor, these decisions are frequent.

They make them multiple times a day—across different patients, different conditions, and different levels of urgency. Over time, the process becomes structured. Clinical reasoning takes shape. Patterns are recognized. Decisions are made with increasing efficiency.

But frequency does not reduce significance.

Each decision carries its own weight, even if it is not always felt in the moment. The responsibility does not diminish with repetition; it becomes embedded within the role.

It becomes part of the profession.

What makes this responsibility unique is that it is often exercised under uncertainty. The doctor does not always have complete information. Conditions evolve, responses vary, and outcomes cannot be guaranteed.

Yet the decision cannot be postponed indefinitely.

Action is required, even when certainty is not available.

This creates a distinct form of authority.

The doctor is entrusted with the power to decide—not because they control outcomes, but because they are best positioned to interpret the situation and choose a course of action. This authority is not taken; it is given.

Given by the patient. Given by society.

And it comes with expectation.

The expectation that the decision will be thoughtful. That it will be based on knowledge, experience, and judgment. That it will prioritize the well-being of the patient above all other considerations.

The expectation is silent, but absolute.

What often remains unseen is the internal dimension of this process. The doctor must weigh options, consider risks, anticipate consequences, and commit to a path—knowing that once the decision is made, it cannot always be reversed.

There is no pause button in real life.

Understanding the weight of a decision is not about creating fear or hesitation. It is about recognizing the depth of the role. It is about acknowledging that authority in medicine is not a position of control, but a position of responsibility.

A responsibility carried in every decision, every day.

Because in the end, medicine is not defined by the number of cases handled or the efficiency of systems.

It is defined by moments—quiet, decisive moments—where one human being takes responsibility for guiding another through uncertainty.

And that responsibility carries weight, whether it is seen or not.

13.1 — Authority in Medicine: Given, Not Claimed

Authority in medicine is unlike authority in most other professions.

It is not asserted. It is entrusted.

A doctor does not demand authority from a patient. It is granted the moment a patient chooses to seek help. When someone walks into a clinic, shares their symptoms, and waits for guidance, they are doing more than consulting—they are transferring a degree of control over their own well-being.

This transfer is built on trust.

The patient assumes that the doctor possesses the knowledge, training, and judgment required to understand their condition and guide them appropriately. They reveal personal information, submit to examinations, and often accept recommendations without fully verifying them.

This is not blind faith—it is functional trust.

Society supports this transfer.

Medical degrees, licensing systems, and regulatory frameworks exist to ensure that those who practice medicine meet certain standards. These structures act as a collective assurance that the authority given to doctors is justified.

The system validates the individual.

But at its core, authority still operates at the level of interaction.

In that moment of consultation, the patient is often in a position of vulnerability. They may be in pain, uncertain about their condition, or anxious about the future. This vulnerability naturally shifts the balance of power.

The doctor becomes the stabilizing presence.

It is this imbalance that makes medical authority distinct.

Unlike authority in administrative or corporate settings, where power may be linked to position or hierarchy, medical authority is directly connected to human need. The patient depends on the doctor not just for information, but for direction.

The doctor's words influence decisions.

This influence carries weight.

A recommendation for a test can lead to financial cost and emotional stress. A diagnosis can change how a person sees their own life. A treatment plan can alter daily routines, long-term health, and future possibilities.

Authority, in this context, shapes outcomes.

Importantly, this authority is conditional.

It exists only as long as trust exists. If patients feel unheard, misunderstood, or misled, the authority weakens. Unlike enforced power, medical authority cannot sustain itself without continued credibility.

It must be maintained, not assumed.

This is why the phrase "given, not claimed" matters.

A doctor may hold a degree, occupy a position, and possess expertise, but authority is activated only when the patient accepts it. It is reaffirmed in every interaction—through clarity of thought, quality of decision-making, and integrity of communication.

It is renewed with each case.

Understanding this nature of authority is essential.

It prevents the profession from drifting toward entitlement. It reminds doctors that their position is not a privilege granted permanently, but a responsibility entrusted temporarily—one patient at a time.

Because in medicine, authority does not originate from status.

It originates from trust—and trust is something that must be earned continuously, not assumed once and carried forward indefinitely.

13.2 — Decision Power Under Uncertainty

In medicine, decisions are rarely made in conditions of complete clarity.

Information is often incomplete. Symptoms may be vague, investigations may be inconclusive, and the condition itself may still be evolving. The doctor must act within this uncertainty, not outside it.

This is the reality of clinical practice.

Unlike controlled environments where variables are fixed and outcomes are predictable, real-world medicine presents dynamic situations. A patient may arrive early in the course of a disease, where signs are subtle. Another may present late, with overlapping complications that obscure the original problem.

The picture is rarely complete.

Yet the decision cannot wait.

Doctors are required to interpret available information, identify the most likely possibilities, and choose a course of action. This involves evaluating probabilities rather than certainties—what is most likely happening, what could happen next, and what intervention is appropriate at that stage.

The process is analytical, but not absolute.

Risk–benefit evaluation becomes central.

Every decision carries potential benefits and potential risks. Starting a treatment may help control a condition, but it may also introduce side effects. Ordering additional tests may provide clarity, but it may also increase cost, time, and anxiety.

The doctor must balance these factors.

In many cases, there is no option that is entirely safe or entirely certain. The doctor must select the option that offers the best possible outcome within the given circumstances.

This is judgment in action.

Time pressure adds another layer of complexity.

In emergencies, decisions must be made quickly, often with limited information. Delaying action to gather more data may increase risk, while acting too early may lead to unnecessary interventions.

The margin for timing is narrow.

Even in non-emergency situations, time influences decision-making. Conditions change, patient responses evolve, and the window for effective intervention may shift. The doctor must continuously reassess and adjust their approach.

Decision-making is not a single event—it is a process.

This process often involves iteration.

An initial diagnosis may be provisional. Treatment may begin with a working hypothesis. As new information becomes available—through patient response, additional tests, or clinical observation—the doctor refines the diagnosis and modifies the plan.

The path is adjusted step by step.

Patients, however, may expect definitive answers.

They may assume that the doctor should know exactly what is happening and what will happen next. When doctors express uncertainty or use terms like "likely," "possible," or "we will monitor," it may be perceived as hesitation.

But it reflects the nature of the field.

Uncertainty in medicine is not a weakness—it is an inherent characteristic. Recognizing it allows doctors to remain cautious, adaptable, and open to revision.

Ignoring it can lead to overconfidence and error.

This is where the responsibility of authority becomes most visible.

The doctor must make decisions that affect outcomes, even when certainty is not available. They must communicate these decisions clearly, manage expectations, and remain accountable for the process.

Authority operates within uncertainty.

Understanding this dynamic is essential for both doctors and patients.

For doctors, it reinforces the need for careful judgment and continuous reassessment. For patients, it helps align expectations with the realities of medical decision-making.

Because in medicine, the absence of certainty does not remove the need for action.

It defines the conditions under which action must be taken.

13.3 — The Ethical Core of Medical Authority

If authority in medicine is granted through trust, then ethics is what sustains it.

Without ethics, authority becomes power. With ethics, authority becomes responsibility.

At the center of medical practice lies a simple but demanding principle: the patient comes first. This principle is easy to state, but difficult to apply consistently, especially in complex situations where multiple factors are at play.

Ethics begins where convenience ends.

A doctor's decision must be guided not by what is easiest, fastest, or most beneficial to the system, but by what is most appropriate for the patient. This includes choosing the right treatment, avoiding unnecessary interventions, and being honest about limitations.

The patient is not a variable. The patient is the purpose.

Two foundational ideas define this ethical core: *beneficence* and *non-maleficence*.

Beneficence requires the doctor to act in the best interest of the patient—to promote well-being, relieve suffering, and support recovery. Non-maleficence requires the doctor to avoid causing harm—whether through action or inaction.

Together, they form a balance.

In practice, this balance is not always straightforward. A treatment that offers potential benefit may also carry risk. A decision to intervene may prevent deterioration but may also introduce complications. The doctor must weigh these possibilities carefully.

Ethics operates within judgment.

Integrity is another essential component.

Doctors must make decisions based on clinical reasoning, not external influences. Financial incentives, institutional pressures, or personal convenience should not alter the course of treatment. When such factors begin to influence decisions, the ethical foundation weakens.

Integrity protects the decision.

Transparency also plays a critical role.

Patients have the right to understand their condition, the available options, and the potential outcomes. Ethical practice requires clear communication—not only about what is being done, but why it is being done. This includes discussing uncertainties and possible risks.

Clarity supports trust.

Confidentiality is another dimension of ethics.

Patients share personal and sensitive information with the expectation that it will be respected and protected. Maintaining confidentiality is not only a legal obligation but also an ethical one, reinforcing the trust that underpins the doctor–patient relationship.

Trust depends on discretion.

Respect for patient autonomy must also be maintained.

While doctors hold expertise, patients have the right to make informed decisions about their own care. Ethical practice involves guiding patients, presenting options, and respecting their choices—even when those choices differ from the doctor's recommendation.

Authority must not override autonomy.

In complex situations, ethical dilemmas can arise.

There may be conflicts between what is medically ideal and what is practically possible. Financial limitations, cultural beliefs, or family dynamics may influence decisions. The doctor must navigate these situations carefully, balancing ideal principles with real-world constraints.

Ethics adapts, but does not disappear.

What makes the ethical core of medical authority unique is that it operates continuously.

It is present in every decision—small or large. Whether it is prescribing a medication, ordering a test, or communicating a diagnosis, ethics shapes the approach and the outcome.

It is not an occasional consideration. It is a constant guide.

Ultimately, the authority given to doctors is justified only when it is exercised ethically.

Because knowledge and skill can create capability, but ethics ensures that capability is used in the right direction.

And in a profession where decisions affect human life, direction matters as much as ability.

13.4 — The Invisible Consequences of Decisions

In medicine, the outcome of a decision is often measured in clinical terms—improvement, stability, complication, or decline.

But the true impact of a medical decision extends far beyond these visible markers.

A diagnosis does not just identify a disease; it changes how a person sees themselves. A label—chronic illness, condition, disorder—can influence identity, behavior, and even relationships. The patient begins to reorganize their life around that understanding.

The consequence is psychological, not just biological.

A treatment plan does not only address symptoms; it alters daily living.

Medications may require long-term adherence, dietary changes may restrict habits, follow-up visits may disrupt routines, and side effects may affect comfort and functioning. What appears as a clinical recommendation becomes a lived experience.

The consequence is practical.

Financial impact is another dimension.

Tests, treatments, hospital stays, and long-term care can create significant economic pressure, especially in systems where healthcare costs are substantial. A decision to proceed with a particular intervention may bring medical benefit but also financial strain.

The consequence is economic.

Family dynamics are often affected.

When a patient becomes dependent—temporarily or permanently—family members adjust their roles. Responsibilities shift, time is redistributed, and emotional stress may increase. Decisions taken in the clinic ripple outward into the patient's immediate environment.

The consequence is relational.

Even the timing of a decision carries implications.

A delayed diagnosis may prolong suffering or complicate treatment. An early intervention may prevent deterioration but may also introduce unnecessary procedures if the condition evolves differently. The sequence of actions shapes the trajectory of outcomes.

The consequence is temporal.

What makes these consequences "invisible" is that they are not always immediately apparent.

A treatment may be clinically successful, yet the patient may struggle with lifestyle adjustments. A correct diagnosis may bring clarity, but also anxiety. A necessary intervention may resolve a condition, but leave lasting emotional or financial effects.

Success is not always simple.

For the doctor, these layers are not always fully visible in the moment of decision.

The focus is often on addressing the immediate clinical problem—identifying the disease, selecting the appropriate treatment, and managing risk. The broader consequences unfold over time, beyond the consultation.

The impact extends beyond the point of care.

This does not imply that doctors must control all outcomes—they cannot. But it highlights the importance of awareness. Recognizing that each decision has multiple dimensions encourages a more thoughtful approach.

Decisions become more holistic.

Communication becomes crucial in this context.

When patients are informed not only about the clinical aspects but also about possible lifestyle, financial, and emotional implications, they are better prepared to navigate the process. This shared understanding reduces surprises and builds trust.

Awareness supports adaptation.

It also reinforces the ethical dimension of authority.

A doctor who considers these broader consequences is not only treating a condition but engaging with the patient's life as a whole. The decision is no longer confined to a clinical outcome—it becomes part of a larger human context.

The role expands.

Understanding invisible consequences does not make decisions easier, but it makes them more grounded. It aligns clinical action with real-world impact, ensuring that treatment is not only effective but also considerate of the patient's overall situation.

Because in medicine, the visible outcome is only part of the story.

The rest unfolds quietly—in the patient's life, long after the decision has been made.

13.5 — Authority Versus Power

In medicine, the line between authority and power is subtle—but critically important.

Authority is grounded in responsibility. Power, when misunderstood, can drift toward control.

A doctor holds a position where their words influence decisions, their recommendations guide actions, and their presence often shapes the emotional state of the patient. This influence is natural, even necessary, because patients seek direction in moments of uncertainty.

But influence must remain aligned with purpose.

Authority in medicine exists to serve the patient. It is exercised through careful judgment, clear communication, and ethical intent. It is limited by the boundaries of knowledge, the autonomy of the patient, and the responsibility to act in their best interest.

It is functional, not dominant.

Power, on the other hand, begins to emerge when this balance shifts.

When a doctor assumes that their position grants unquestionable control, when patient input is dismissed, or when decisions are imposed without explanation, authority starts to transform into power. The interaction becomes less collaborative and more hierarchical.

The relationship changes.

This shift is not always intentional.

It can arise from habit, workload, or the structure of the system itself. In busy environments, where time is limited and decisions must be made quickly, communication may become brief, and patient involvement may reduce. Over time, this can create a pattern where decisions are delivered rather than discussed.

Efficiency begins to override engagement.

In some cases, the perception of expertise can contribute to this dynamic.

Doctors are trained extensively and are expected to lead clinical decision-making. This expectation can, at times, create a sense of certainty that discourages questioning—both from the doctor and from the patient.

Confidence, if unchecked, can become rigidity.

The risk here is not only ethical but practical.

When authority becomes power, valuable information may be lost. Patients may hesitate to share concerns, ask questions, or express doubts. This reduces the quality of interaction and can affect the accuracy of diagnosis and the effectiveness of treatment.

Silence replaces participation.

Trust is also affected.

Patients are more likely to trust doctors who explain, listen, and involve them in decisions. When they feel excluded or overridden, even correct decisions may be perceived negatively. The relationship becomes transactional rather than collaborative.

Trust weakens when voice is removed.

It is important to recognize that authority and power are not the same.

Authority is granted because of expertise and maintained through ethical use. Power is perceived when that authority is exercised without alignment to the patient's perspective. The distinction lies not in the position, but in how it is used.

Intent defines direction.

Maintaining this distinction requires awareness.

Doctors must remain conscious of how their decisions are communicated, how much space is given for patient input, and whether their approach encourages understanding or simply enforces compliance.

Awareness prevents drift.

Respect for patient autonomy plays a key role.

While doctors provide expertise, patients retain the right to make informed choices about their own care. Supporting this autonomy does not weaken authority—it strengthens it by building trust and cooperation.

Shared decision-making reinforces alignment.

Ultimately, the goal is not to eliminate authority, but to preserve its purpose.

A doctor must lead when necessary, decide when required, and guide with clarity. But this leadership must remain rooted in responsibility, not control.

Because in medicine, authority is not a tool for dominance.

It is a responsibility to guide another human being through uncertainty—with knowledge, integrity, and respect.

13.6 — External Pressures on Medical Decisions

In principle, medical decisions should emerge from a clear foundation—clinical knowledge, patient context, and ethical judgment.

In practice, the decision environment is rarely that pure.

Doctors today operate within systems that introduce multiple external pressures. These pressures are not always visible to patients, but they influence how decisions are shaped, communicated, and executed.

The clinical space is no longer isolated.

One of the most significant pressures comes from institutional structures.

Hospitals and healthcare organizations function as complex systems with operational requirements. Patient flow must be managed, resources must be allocated, and efficiency must be maintained. Doctors working within these systems often need to align with protocols, schedules, and performance expectations.

The decision exists within a framework.

This framework is not inherently negative—it enables organized care and scalability. But when operational priorities begin to intersect with clinical judgment, subtle tensions can arise. Time constraints may limit detailed discussions. Standardized pathways may not fully accommodate individual variation.

The system introduces boundaries.

Financial factors add another layer.

Healthcare, especially in private settings, involves significant cost structures. Decisions about investigations, procedures, and treatment plans may intersect with considerations of affordability, insurance coverage, and institutional economics.

The doctor must navigate both care and cost.

This creates complex situations.

A clinically ideal option may not always be financially feasible for the patient. Conversely, the availability of advanced interventions may encourage their use even when simpler alternatives could suffice. Balancing medical appropriateness with economic reality requires careful judgment.

The decision extends beyond medicine.

Legal considerations also play a major role.

Medical practice is increasingly subject to scrutiny. Doctors must be aware that their decisions can be questioned in legal contexts. Documentation, consent, and adherence to guidelines become critical, not only for patient care but also for protection against potential disputes.

Every decision carries legal visibility.

This awareness can influence behavior.

Doctors may adopt defensive practices—ordering additional tests, avoiding high-risk decisions, or strictly adhering to protocols—to minimize exposure to legal risk. While this can provide protection, it may also affect the efficiency and personalization of care.

Caution becomes part of the process.

Social and reputational factors contribute as well.

In an interconnected world, patient experiences are shared widely. Public perception, reviews, and community narratives can influence how doctors approach communication and decision-making. The need to maintain credibility adds another dimension to professional responsibility.

Perception begins to matter alongside outcome.

Workload is another significant pressure.

High patient volumes, long working hours, and continuous responsibility can affect cognitive clarity and emotional balance. Under such conditions, maintaining optimal decision-making consistently becomes more challenging.

The human system is under strain.

What makes these pressures particularly complex is that they often operate simultaneously.

A doctor may need to make a decision that is clinically sound, financially feasible, legally defensible, institutionally aligned, and communicatively acceptable—all within limited time.

The decision becomes multidimensional.

This does not mean that external pressures dictate decisions, but they inevitably influence the environment in which decisions are made. Recognizing their presence is important, both for doctors and for patients.

Awareness creates context.

For doctors, it reinforces the need to remain anchored in clinical judgment and ethical principles, even when navigating these pressures. For patients, it provides a more complete understanding of the factors that shape medical care.

Because medicine does not operate in isolation.

It operates within systems—and those systems, while necessary, introduce complexities that extend beyond the clinical condition itself.

13.7 — Owning the Outcome

Authority in medicine reaches its true meaning not at the moment of decision, but after it.

When the outcome unfolds.

Every medical decision sets a process in motion. The patient responds, the condition evolves, and results begin to appear—sometimes as expected, sometimes differently. At this stage, the role of the doctor does not end. It transforms.

From decision-maker to owner of the outcome.

Owning the outcome does not mean controlling it completely—that is neither possible nor realistic. Medicine operates within uncertainty, and not all variables can be predicted or managed. But ownership means remaining connected to the consequence of the decision.

It means not stepping away once the action is taken.

When outcomes are positive, ownership may appear simple. The treatment works, the patient improves, and the process seems validated. But even here, true ownership involves reflection—understanding why the decision worked, reinforcing the reasoning, and learning from the success.

Success, too, requires awareness.

The real test of ownership, however, appears when outcomes are not as expected.

A treatment may not produce the desired effect. Complications may arise. A diagnosis may need revision. In such situations, the doctor must remain engaged—reassessing the case, adapting the approach, and communicating clearly with the patient.

Ownership means staying present in difficulty.

It also requires honesty.

Explaining outcomes—whether favorable or unfavorable—demands clarity and transparency. Patients may not always accept the result, but they are more likely to trust a process where the doctor communicates openly and takes responsibility for guiding the next steps.

Clarity sustains trust.

Accountability is a key component of ownership.

This does not imply blame for every negative outcome. Medicine involves factors beyond control. But it does mean acknowledging the decision, reviewing its reasoning, and accepting responsibility for the role played in the process.

Accountability builds integrity.

Reflection transforms ownership into growth.

Each outcome, whether successful or not, provides insight. What assumptions were made? What variables were considered? What could be improved in future decisions? This reflective process refines judgment and strengthens future practice.

Experience becomes intelligence.

Humility plays an important role.

Doctors must recognize that even with knowledge and skill, errors or unexpected outcomes can occur. Accepting this reality does not weaken authority—it makes it more grounded. It prevents overconfidence and encourages continuous learning.

Humility protects judgment.

Ownership also extends to continuity of care.

Following up with patients, adjusting treatment plans, and ensuring that the patient remains supported throughout the process reinforces the doctor's commitment. It shows that the decision was not an isolated act, but part of an ongoing responsibility.

Care continues beyond action.

In systems where workload is high and interactions are brief, maintaining this sense of ownership can be challenging. But even small actions—reviewing outcomes, checking progress, communicating updates—help sustain the connection between decision and consequence.

Responsibility is expressed through continuity.

Ultimately, owning the outcome is what distinguishes authority from mere action.

Anyone can make a decision. Not everyone stays with its consequences.

In medicine, staying matters.

Because for the patient, the outcome is not a case—it is their life. And the doctor who remains engaged with that outcome, learns from it, and continues to guide the process embodies the true responsibility of authority.

Not as a moment of control, but as a commitment that extends beyond the decision itself.

Authority as Responsibility, Not Privilege

Authority in medicine is often visible on the surface.

It appears in the white coat, in the prescription, in the final word that guides the course of treatment. It is seen in the confidence with which decisions are made and in the trust that patients place without fully understanding the complexity behind those decisions.

From the outside, it can look like privilege.

But from within, it feels different.

It feels like weight.

A weight that is carried quietly, without display. A weight that does not reduce with experience, but becomes more refined. With every patient, every decision, every outcome, the awareness deepens—not of power, but of responsibility.

Because authority in medicine is not ownership of control.

It is acceptance of consequence.

A doctor does not control how a body responds, how a disease progresses, or how an outcome unfolds. What they control is the decision they make within that moment—the reasoning behind it, the care with which it is applied, and the integrity with which it is communicated.

The authority lies in that choice.

And with that choice comes responsibility—not only for the immediate action, but for its ripple effects. For the patient's experience, for their trust, for the path that unfolds after the decision.

This is not a privilege that elevates.

It is a responsibility that grounds.

It demands clarity in thinking, restraint in action, and honesty in communication. It requires the doctor to remain aligned with purpose, even when external pressures exist, even when outcomes are uncertain, even when recognition is absent.

Because responsibility does not depend on visibility.

It exists whether it is acknowledged or not.

In modern medicine, where systems are complex and expectations are high, it is easy to confuse authority with status. But status can be claimed. Authority, in its true sense, must be justified continuously—through decisions, through conduct, through consistency.

It must be lived, not displayed.

When authority is understood as responsibility, the nature of practice changes.

Decisions become more thoughtful. Communication becomes more transparent. Interactions become more respectful. The doctor does not stand above the patient, but alongside them—guiding, not controlling.

The relationship becomes balanced.

This perspective does not reduce the importance of the doctor's role—it clarifies it. It brings the focus back to what matters: the application of knowledge with integrity, the use of judgment with care, and the acceptance of responsibility for the path chosen.

Because in the end, authority in medicine is not about having the right to decide.

It is about being ready to carry the weight of that decision.

And that weight—when carried with awareness—is what defines the true meaning of being a doctor.

Chapter 14 — What It Truly Means to Be a Doctor

Beyond the Role

After everything that has been discussed—the system, the pressures, the expectations, the distortions—a simple question remains:

What does it truly mean to be a doctor?

Not in definition. Not in qualification. But in practice.

Because somewhere along the way, the role has become layered.

Medicine is now a system. Healthcare is an industry. Doctors are professionals within structured environments.

There are protocols to follow, targets to meet, documentation to maintain, and expectations to manage. The role is defined externally—by institutions, by regulations, by society.

But beneath all of this, there is something more fundamental.

A doctor is not created by the system alone.

The system can train, certify, and position an individual. It can provide knowledge, exposure, and structure. But it cannot fully define what the doctor becomes in practice.

That definition emerges from within.

It emerges in how decisions are made when no one is watching. In how a patient is treated when time is limited. In how responsibility is carried when outcomes are uncertain.

The role is lived, not assigned.

Modern medicine has created complexity, but it has also created distance.

Distance between doctor and patient. Distance between knowledge and application. Distance between role and purpose.

This distance is not always visible, but it is often felt.

Patients feel it when interactions become mechanical. Doctors feel it when practice becomes routine. The system feels it when trust begins to weaken.

And yet, the essence of medicine has not changed.

At its core, it remains one human being applying knowledge and judgment to help another human being navigate illness. This interaction is simple, but the environment around it has become complex.

The challenge today is not to simplify the system.

It is to remain clear within it.

To practice science without losing humanity. To carry authority without losing responsibility. To function within systems without becoming defined by them.

This requires a conscious redefinition.

Not imposed from outside, but chosen from within.

Because being a doctor today is not just about meeting standards—it is about maintaining balance. Balance between what is known and what is uncertain. Between what is required and what is right. Between efficiency and care.

This balance defines the profession.

And perhaps that is where the true meaning lies—not in the title, not in the degree, not in the system—but in the ability to remain aligned with the purpose of medicine, even as everything around it continues to change.

That is the doctor we now need to rediscover.

14.1 — The Three Pillars: Science, Humanity, Responsibility

To understand what it truly means to be a doctor, the profession must be viewed through three essential pillars:

Science. Humanity. Responsibility.

Individually, each is important. Together, they define the profession.

Science is the foundation.

Medicine begins with knowledge—the structured understanding of the human body, disease mechanisms, diagnostics, and treatment. Without science, there is no accuracy, no direction, and no ability to intervene effectively.

Science provides clarity.

It allows doctors to identify patterns, interpret findings, and apply treatments that are based on evidence rather than assumption. It is what differentiates medicine from guesswork. It gives the profession its intellectual strength and credibility.

But science alone is not sufficient.

Because science deals with systems. Medicine deals with people.

Humanity is the connection.

A patient is not a biological problem to be solved. They are a person experiencing discomfort, fear, uncertainty, and often vulnerability. Their condition affects not only their body but their emotions, their relationships, and their sense of stability.

Humanity allows the doctor to see this.

It is reflected in listening carefully, speaking clearly, and responding with empathy. It is present in the tone of explanation, in the patience shown during consultation, and in the ability to make the patient feel understood.

Humanity builds trust.

Without it, even the most accurate treatment can feel incomplete. Patients may follow instructions, but they may not feel supported. The interaction becomes functional rather than meaningful.

And medicine, at its core, is more than function.

Responsibility is the direction.

Authority in medicine gives the doctor the power to make decisions. Responsibility ensures that this power is used correctly. It aligns knowledge and action with purpose.

Responsibility defines intent.

It requires the doctor to act in the best interest of the patient, to remain honest about uncertainties, and to stay accountable for decisions and outcomes. It ensures that science is applied ethically and humanity is sustained consistently.

Responsibility carries weight.

It is present in every prescription written, every diagnosis communicated, and every decision made under pressure. It does not disappear when the consultation ends—it continues through follow-up, reflection, and ongoing care.

These three pillars are not independent.

Science without humanity becomes mechanical. Humanity without science becomes ineffective. Both without responsibility become unstable.

Balance is essential.

A doctor grounded only in science may treat disease but miss the person. A doctor guided only by empathy may connect well but lack clinical precision. A doctor without a sense of responsibility may possess both knowledge and compassion but fail to align them with consistent action.

The profession requires integration.

In modern healthcare, where systems are complex and pressures are high, maintaining this balance becomes more challenging. Time constraints may reduce human connection. Institutional demands may influence responsibility. Information overload may complicate scientific clarity.

The pillars are tested continuously.

Yet, it is this very balance that defines the doctor.

Not the degree. Not the system. Not the title.

But the ability to integrate science, humanity, and responsibility into a single, coherent way of practicing medicine.

Because when these three pillars align, medicine regains its essence.

And the doctor becomes not just a professional within a system, but a complete practitioner of a discipline that exists at the intersection of knowledge and life.

14.2 — From Treatment to Care

Modern medicine is highly effective at treating disease.

It can diagnose with precision, intervene with advanced techniques, and manage conditions with structured protocols. The system is designed to identify problems and apply solutions.

This is treatment.

But treatment, by itself, is only a part of what patients actually need.

Because a patient does not arrive with a disease alone. They arrive with an experience.

An experience of discomfort, fear, confusion, and uncertainty. An experience shaped by family expectations, financial concerns, social identity, and personal resilience. The disease may be the clinical focus, but the experience is what the patient lives through.

Care begins where treatment ends.

Treatment focuses on the condition. Care includes the person.

When a doctor shifts from treating to caring, the interaction changes.

The consultation is no longer limited to identifying symptoms and prescribing solutions. It expands to understanding how the condition affects the patient's life—how it disrupts routines, alters emotions, and creates uncertainty about the future.

The conversation becomes broader.

A patient with a chronic condition is not just managing symptoms—they are adjusting their lifestyle. A patient undergoing surgery is not just facing a procedure—they are dealing with fear and dependency. A patient receiving a diagnosis is not just receiving information—they are processing a shift in their identity.

Care acknowledges these layers.

Listening becomes a clinical skill.

In treatment-driven interactions, listening is often focused—directed toward extracting relevant symptoms and medical history. In care-driven interactions, listening expands to include context.

What is the patient worried about? What are they not saying directly? What constraints are they facing outside the clinic?

These questions are not separate from medicine—they are part of it.

Because understanding the patient's context improves decision-making. It helps tailor treatment plans that are realistic, acceptable, and sustainable. It reduces non-compliance not through enforcement, but through alignment.

Listening improves outcomes.

Communication becomes part of treatment.

In care-oriented practice, what the doctor says—and how it is said—matters as much as the prescription itself.

Clear explanations reduce anxiety. Transparent discussions build trust. Realistic expectations prevent disappointment.

Patients are more likely to follow a plan they understand. They are more likely to cooperate when they feel respected. Communication is not an additional step—it is an integral part of effective care.

Words influence healing.

Continuity defines care.

Treatment can be episodic—a consultation, a procedure, a prescription. Care is continuous.

It involves follow-up, reassessment, and adjustment. It recognizes that conditions evolve, responses vary, and patient circumstances change over time.

Care stays with the patient.

Even small acts—checking progress, adjusting medication, addressing new concerns—reinforce this continuity. They signal that the doctor's role is not limited to a moment, but extends across the patient's journey.

Continuity builds confidence.

Care does not mean more time—it means better alignment.

A common assumption is that caring requires significantly more time. In reality, it requires better use of time.

A focused conversation that addresses both the clinical issue and the patient's concerns can prevent repeated visits, misunderstandings, and non-compliance. It can reduce friction in the system and improve efficiency in the long run.

Care is not inefficiency. It is intelligent practice.

The shift is subtle, but powerful.

Moving from treatment to care does not require abandoning science or protocols. It requires expanding the perspective.

The disease remains important. But the person becomes central.

When this shift occurs, medicine becomes more than intervention—it becomes engagement. The doctor is no longer just solving a problem, but guiding a process.

And the patient is no longer just receiving treatment, but participating in their own recovery.

Because in the end, patients may forget the technical details of their treatment.

But they rarely forget how they were treated as human beings.

And that difference—between treatment and care—is what defines the true practice of medicine.

14.3 — The Doctor as a Stabilizing Presence

Illness introduces instability.

It disrupts the body, unsettles the mind, and often creates uncertainty across the patient's life. Decisions become difficult, information feels overwhelming, and emotions begin to fluctuate—fear, anxiety, doubt.

In that moment, the patient is not just seeking treatment.

They are seeking stability.

The doctor becomes the point of reference.

When a patient enters the clinical space, they are entering a system they do not fully understand. Medical language is unfamiliar, processes are complex, and outcomes are uncertain.

The doctor becomes the anchor in this environment.

Not because they have all the answers, but because they provide direction. Their presence offers a sense of order in a situation that feels disorganized. Their clarity helps reduce confusion. Their confidence helps reduce fear.

Stability begins with presence.

Confidence without arrogance.

A stabilizing presence requires confidence—but not dominance.

Patients need to feel that the doctor understands the situation and is capable of guiding the process. This confidence comes from knowledge, experience, and clarity in thinking.

But when confidence turns into arrogance, stability is lost.

Arrogance creates distance. It discourages questions, reduces openness, and can make patients feel dismissed. Confidence, when balanced with humility, invites engagement and builds trust.

The difference is subtle, but critical.

Clarity in communication.

Uncertainty increases when communication is unclear.

Patients may receive complex explanations, technical terms, or fragmented information that adds to their confusion. A stabilizing doctor translates complexity into clarity.

What is the condition? What are the options? What is likely to happen next?

When these questions are answered clearly, the patient regains a sense of control. They may still be uncertain about the outcome, but they understand the path.

Clarity reduces chaos.

Calm in critical moments.

In emergency or high-pressure situations, the doctor's behavior directly influences the environment.

A calm approach can stabilize not only the patient, but also the family and even the healthcare team. It signals that the situation is being managed, even when it is serious.

Panic spreads quickly. So does calm.

Maintaining composure does not mean ignoring the seriousness of the situation—it means responding to it in a controlled and focused manner.

Calm supports decision-making.

Guiding, not controlling.

A stabilizing presence does not override the patient—it guides them.

Patients and families often look for direction, but they also need to feel involved. The doctor's role is to present options, explain implications, and help them navigate choices.

This creates a collaborative dynamic.

When patients feel guided rather than controlled, they are more likely to trust the process and participate actively. Stability is not imposed—it is shared.

Participation strengthens stability.

Consistency builds reliability.

Stability is not created in a single interaction—it is built over time.

Consistent behavior, consistent communication, and consistent decision-making patterns reinforce trust. Patients begin to understand how the doctor approaches situations, and this predictability reduces anxiety.

Reliability creates comfort.

Even in uncertain outcomes, a consistent approach provides a stable framework within which patients can operate.

Stability extends beyond the individual patient.

The doctor's role as a stabilizing presence is not limited to one interaction.

It influences the broader system.

Families rely on the doctor's guidance. Healthcare teams align with the doctor's decisions. The overall environment of care becomes more structured when the doctor maintains clarity and composure.

One stable node affects the entire system.

The deeper role of the doctor.

When viewed from this perspective, the doctor is not just a provider of treatment.

They are a stabilizing force within a dynamic and often uncertain system.

They absorb complexity, filter it through knowledge and judgment, and present it in a form that others can understand and act upon.

They reduce uncertainty—not by eliminating it, but by making it manageable.

Because in moments of illness, what patients often need most is not certainty.

It is someone who can stand steady within uncertainty.

And that steadiness—that ability to remain clear, calm, and responsible—is what defines the doctor as a stabilizing presence.

14.4 — Rebuilding Trust in Modern Medicine

Trust in medicine was once assumed.

A doctor's word was accepted without hesitation. Decisions were followed without question. The relationship between doctor and patient operated on an implicit understanding—one guided by respect, belief, and reliance.

Today, that trust is no longer automatic.

It must be earned.

The shift from blind trust to informed trust.

Patients today are more informed, more aware, and more questioning. Access to information—accurate or otherwise—has changed how people approach healthcare. They arrive with prior opinions, online research, and sometimes conflicting inputs.

This has transformed the dynamic.

Trust is no longer based on position alone. It is based on interaction.

Patients now evaluate not just what the doctor knows, but how the doctor communicates, explains, and involves them in decisions.

Trust has become active.

Transparency as a foundation.

In this environment, transparency becomes essential.

Patients need to understand not only the diagnosis and treatment, but also the reasoning behind decisions. When doctors explain the "why" along with the "what," they reduce ambiguity and build confidence.

Transparency does not require oversimplification—it requires clarity.

It includes discussing uncertainties, potential risks, and alternative approaches. It acknowledges that medicine is not always absolute, and that decisions are often made within a range of possibilities.

Honesty strengthens credibility.

Consistency in practice.

Trust is reinforced when behavior is consistent.

If a doctor communicates clearly in one interaction but appears dismissive in another, the inconsistency creates doubt. Patients begin to question reliability, even if the clinical decisions are correct.

Consistency creates predictability.

When patients know what to expect—in terms of communication, approach, and conduct—they feel more secure. This stability supports trust, especially in long-term care relationships.

Reliability builds confidence.

Ethical clarity in decisions.

Trust is also influenced by perceived intent.

Patients are sensitive to whether decisions are being made in their best interest or influenced by external factors. Even the perception of financial or institutional bias can weaken trust, regardless of the actual reasoning.

Intent must be visible.

When doctors clearly align decisions with patient benefit—avoiding unnecessary interventions, explaining cost considerations honestly, and prioritizing clinical appropriateness—trust is reinforced.

Ethics becomes observable.

Communication during uncertainty.

Trust is most fragile when outcomes are uncertain or unfavorable.

In such situations, silence or avoidance can quickly erode confidence. Patients need guidance, even when answers are not definitive. They need to understand what is happening, what is being done, and what can be expected next.

Presence matters more than certainty.

A doctor who communicates openly during difficult moments—acknowledging uncertainty while providing direction—maintains trust even in challenging situations.

Respect as a constant.

Trust is not built only through decisions—it is built through interaction.

Simple elements—listening attentively, addressing concerns without dismissal, and treating patients with dignity—play a significant role. Respect is perceived immediately and remembered consistently.

Respect humanizes the interaction.

When patients feel respected, they are more likely to trust—even when they disagree or do not fully understand the medical details.

Shared responsibility in trust.

Rebuilding trust is not the responsibility of doctors alone.

Patients also play a role—by engaging honestly, providing accurate information, and approaching interactions with openness rather than assumption. Trust is a two-way process, shaped by both sides.

The relationship is mutual.

Trust as a continuous process.

Trust is not established in a single consultation.

It develops over time—through repeated interactions, consistent behavior, and transparent communication. It can be strengthened gradually or weakened quickly.

It requires maintenance.

In modern medicine, where systems are complex and expectations are high, trust becomes one of the most critical elements of effective care.

Because without trust, even the best decisions may be questioned. And with trust, even difficult decisions can be accepted.

Rebuilding trust is not about returning to the past.

It is about adapting to the present.

Creating a model where knowledge is combined with communication, authority is balanced with transparency, and decisions are aligned with visible intent.

Because in the end, trust is not given to the profession.

It is given to the person practicing it.

And that trust—once built—becomes the strongest foundation of modern medicine.

14.5 — Practicing Medicine Without Losing Self

Medicine demands a great deal from those who practice it.

Time, attention, emotional energy, intellectual rigor, and constant responsibility—these are not occasional requirements; they are continuous. Over time, this demand can begin to reshape the individual behind the profession.

The doctor becomes the role.

And somewhere in that process, the person risks fading.

The quiet erosion of self.

The journey to becoming a doctor is long and consuming. Years of study, training, and exposure to suffering gradually condition the mind to operate in a certain way—focused, efficient, and often emotionally restrained.

This conditioning is necessary.

But when it extends unchecked into everyday life, it begins to erode the individual's natural balance. Conversations become clinical, emotions become controlled, and personal experiences are filtered through professional logic.

The boundary blurs.

Emotional detachment as a default state.

To function effectively, doctors often develop a level of emotional detachment. It allows them to make decisions without being overwhelmed, to handle repeated exposure to illness, and to maintain clarity under pressure.

This detachment is protective.

But when it becomes habitual, it can extend beyond the clinical environment. The doctor may begin to feel distant not only from patients, but also from family, friends, and even their own internal experiences.

Protection turns into isolation.

The risk of identity collapse.

When professional identity dominates completely, other aspects of the self receive less attention.

Interests outside medicine diminish. Personal relationships may weaken. The individual's sense of self becomes tightly linked to their role as a doctor.

This creates vulnerability.

Because when challenges arise within the profession—stress, failure, criticism, or burnout—the impact is not limited to the role. It affects the entire identity.

The self becomes dependent on the profession.

The need for conscious separation.

To sustain long-term practice, doctors must maintain a clear distinction between who they are and what they do.

The role is important. But it is not the entirety of the person.

Creating this separation does not reduce commitment—it preserves it. It allows the doctor to return to their work with clarity, rather than exhaustion. It provides space for recovery, reflection, and renewal.

Separation supports continuity.

Personal boundaries as professional strength.

Setting boundaries is often misunderstood as disengagement. In reality, it is a form of discipline.

Boundaries define when the doctor is fully present in their role and when they step back to restore balance. They protect against overextension, reduce the risk of burnout, and help maintain consistent performance over time.

Boundaries sustain capacity.

A doctor who is constantly stretched beyond limits may continue to function temporarily, but the quality of decisions, communication, and care eventually declines.

Sustainability matters.

Meaning beyond routine.

Over time, repetitive exposure to similar cases and processes can create a sense of routine. The work may become predictable, and the initial sense of purpose may begin to fade.

This is a critical point.

Doctors must reconnect with the meaning of their work—not through external recognition, but through internal alignment. Recognizing the impact of their role, even in small interactions, helps maintain a sense of purpose.

Meaning restores engagement.

Regular reflection allows doctors to recalibrate.

What decisions were made today? What interactions felt aligned or misaligned? What can be improved?

This process is not about self-criticism—it is about awareness. It helps maintain clarity, prevents drift, and supports continuous growth.

Reflection maintains direction.

A doctor who preserves their sense of self is not less committed—they are more effective.

They communicate better because they are emotionally available. They decide better because they are mentally clear. They sustain longer because they are not continuously depleted.

Balance enhances performance.

Practicing medicine without losing self is not about reducing responsibility.

It is about managing it intelligently.

It is about recognizing that the doctor is not just a function within a system, but a human being operating within demanding conditions.

And preserving that humanity—within oneself—is what ultimately allows the doctor to offer it to others.

Because a doctor who remains whole can care more effectively than one who is gradually fragmented by the very profession they serve.

14.6 — The Evolving Doctor in a Changing System

Medicine is no longer what it was a few decades ago.

The environment has changed—rapidly and irreversibly.

Technology has entered the consultation room. Data flows faster than understanding. Systems are larger, more structured, and more demanding. Patients are more informed, more questioning, and more connected.

The doctor is no longer operating in a static profession.

They are operating in an evolving system.

The rise of technology and data.

Diagnostics are more precise. Imaging is more advanced. Algorithms assist in pattern recognition. Artificial intelligence is beginning to support decision-making processes.

These developments are powerful.

They enhance accuracy, improve efficiency, and expand the possibilities of care. But they also change the role of the doctor.

From being the sole source of knowledge to being an interpreter of knowledge.

The doctor must now evaluate outputs, validate information, and integrate technological insights with clinical judgment.

Technology supports—but does not replace—thinking.

Information overload and decision complexity.

With increased access to data comes increased complexity.

Multiple guidelines, evolving research, and varying interpretations can make decision-making more challenging. The doctor must navigate this information landscape, filter what is relevant, and apply it appropriately to individual cases.

Not all information is equally useful.

Judgment becomes more critical than ever.

The ability to simplify complexity—to identify what truly matters for the patient in front—is what defines effective practice in this environment.

Clarity becomes a skill.

System-driven practice versus individual judgment.

Modern healthcare systems rely on protocols, pathways, and standardization.

These frameworks are necessary. They improve consistency, reduce errors, and enable large-scale delivery of care. But they also introduce a risk.

The risk of over-reliance.

When protocols are followed without thoughtful interpretation, medicine can become mechanical. Individual patient variation may be overlooked. Unique contexts may be forced into standardized models.

The system provides structure. The doctor provides judgment.

Balancing these two is essential.

A good doctor does not reject systems—but neither do they surrender their reasoning to them. They use protocols as tools, not as substitutes for thinking.

Changing patient expectations.

Patients today expect more than treatment.

They expect explanation, involvement, and transparency. They seek clarity about options, risks, and outcomes. They compare information, question decisions, and engage actively in their care.

This is not a challenge—it is an evolution.

It shifts the role of the doctor from authority alone to guide and collaborator. It requires stronger communication, greater patience, and a willingness to engage in dialogue.

The interaction becomes participatory.

Time pressure and efficiency demands.

Despite increasing complexity, time per patient often remains limited.

Doctors must make decisions quickly, communicate effectively, and manage multiple responsibilities simultaneously. This creates tension between depth and efficiency.

The system demands speed. The profession requires thought.

Navigating this tension is one of the defining challenges of modern practice. It requires prioritization, clarity, and the ability to focus on what matters most within limited time.

Efficiency must not eliminate care.

Continuous learning as a necessity.

The pace of change means that knowledge does not remain static.

New treatments emerge. Guidelines evolve. Technologies advance. The doctor must continuously update their understanding—not as an option, but as a requirement.

Learning becomes ongoing.

This is not limited to clinical knowledge. It includes communication skills, ethical awareness, system navigation, and adaptation to new tools.

The evolving doctor is a learning doctor.

Preserving core values within change.

Amid all these shifts, one risk stands out—the dilution of core values.

When systems dominate, when technology becomes central, when efficiency overrides interaction, the foundational elements of medicine can weaken.

This is where conscious effort is required.

To preserve humanity within technology. To maintain responsibility within systems. To uphold ethics within complexity.

The core must remain stable, even as the environment changes.

Adaptation without loss of identity.

The evolving doctor is not someone who resists change.

They adapt—but with awareness.

They integrate new tools without becoming dependent on them. They follow systems without losing judgment. They engage with informed patients without feeling threatened.

They evolve without losing their core.

Because the future of medicine will not be defined only by technology or systems.

It will be defined by how doctors position themselves within them.

Whether they become operators within a system

or remain thoughtful practitioners who use the system intelligently.

The evolving doctor understands one thing clearly:

Change is inevitable. Loss of essence is not.

And the ability to adapt while staying grounded is what will define the true doctor in the years to come.

14.7 — A Personal Definition of Being a Doctor

After all the systems, structures, pressures, and expectations are stripped away, one question remains—quiet, but unavoidable: Who are you as a doctor?

Not what your degree says. Not what your institution expects. Not what society assumes.

But what you choose to be—consistently, in practice.

The profession gives you a role. You define how it is lived.

Medical education provides knowledge. Training provides exposure. Systems provide structure.

But none of these can define your personal standard.

That standard is internal.

It appears in small moments—how you speak to a patient when you are tired, how you respond when questioned, how you decide when options are unclear.

Your definition is expressed through behavior.

Clarity of purpose.

Every doctor begins with a reason—sometimes clear, sometimes shaped over time.

For some, it is intellectual interest. For others, stability, respect, or opportunity. For many, it evolves into responsibility.

At some point, however, the question becomes sharper: Why do I practice medicine the way I do?

Without clarity, practice becomes reactive—driven by system demands, routine, or external pressures. With clarity, decisions gain direction.

Purpose organizes action.

Alignment between belief and action.

A doctor may believe in ethical practice, patient-centered care, and professional responsibility. But the true test lies in alignment.

Do decisions reflect those beliefs? Does behavior remain consistent under pressure?

Misalignment is subtle but significant.

It appears when convenience overrides judgment, when communication is reduced to efficiency, or when responsibility is delegated without reflection.

Alignment requires awareness.

Consistency across situations.

It is easier to act correctly when conditions are ideal.

The real definition of a doctor emerges in less ideal circumstances—when time is limited, when cases are complex, when outcomes are uncertain.

Consistency becomes the measure.

A doctor who maintains clarity, respect, and responsibility across varying conditions builds a stable professional identity.

Consistency builds trust—internally and externally.

Ownership of professional identity.

In modern systems, it is easy to feel that the role is defined externally—by protocols, institutions, or administrative structures.

But ultimately, the doctor must take ownership.

Not of the system—but of how they function within it.

Ownership means making conscious choices:

- How much time to invest in understanding the patient
- How to balance efficiency with care
- How to respond to pressure without compromising integrity

The system influences. The doctor decides.

The role of reflection.

Defining oneself is not a one-time act—it is an ongoing process.

Regular reflection allows adjustment.

What kind of doctor am I becoming? Is this aligned with what I intended? What needs to change?

This process prevents drift.

Without reflection, behavior gradually adapts to convenience or pressure. With reflection, it remains aligned with purpose.

Individual definition within a shared profession.

All doctors share a common foundation—science, training, and responsibility.

But how each doctor practices can vary.

Some may prioritize depth of communication. Some may focus on precision and efficiency. Some may emphasize long-term patient relationships.

There is space for individuality.

But this individuality must remain anchored in core principles—ethics, responsibility, and respect for the patient.

Freedom exists within boundaries.

The quiet power of a defined self.

A doctor who has defined their approach does not need external validation to maintain it.

They are less influenced by shifting expectations, less reactive to pressure, and more consistent in their decisions.

Their practice becomes stable.

Not rigid—but grounded.

Because in the end, medicine is not practiced by systems.

It is practiced by individuals within systems.

And while the system shapes the environment, the doctor shapes the experience.

Your degree made you a doctor. Your definition will decide what kind of doctor you become.

The Doctor the World Needs Today

After everything—training, pressure, systems, expectations—the profession arrives at a quiet but defining realization:

The world does not need more doctors. It needs *clear doctors.* Not just knowledgeable. Not just skilled. But aligned.

We are living in a time where medicine is advancing rapidly. Technology is improving diagnostics. Systems are expanding access. Information is everywhere.

And yet, something feels unsettled. Patients feel unheard. Doctors feel exhausted. Trust feels fragile.

The problem is not a lack of progress. It is a lack of balance.

The doctor the world needs today is not an idealized figure. Not a god. Not a machine. Not a perfect decision-maker. But a *balanced practitioner.*

One who understands science deeply, but does not hide behind it. One who connects with patients, but does not lose clarity. One who carries responsibility, but does not collapse under it.

Balance is the new competence.

This doctor does not try to control everything. They understand that uncertainty is part of medicine. They do not promise certainty—they provide direction. They do not dominate the interaction—they guide it. They do not reduce patients to cases—they engage with them as participants.

They are not driven only by outcomes. They are driven by *process integrity.* Because outcomes can vary. But the way a decision is made, explained, and carried—that remains within control. And that is where trust is built.

They are also aware of themselves. They recognize their limits. They manage their energy. They maintain their identity beyond the profession.

Because a fragmented doctor cannot create a stable system. Only a balanced individual can function as a stabilizing force. In a system full of complexity, this doctor becomes simple.

Clear thinking. Clear communication. Clear intent.

Not simplistic—but clear. And that clarity becomes their strength. This is not a return to the past. It is an evolution.

From authority to responsibility. From treatment to care. From system-driven action to conscious practice.

The future of medicine will not be defined only by innovation.

It will be defined by *how doctors choose to practice within that innovation.*

Whether they become operators or remain thoughtful practitioners. And perhaps that is the final truth:

Being a doctor is not about reaching a standard. It is about *continuously aligning with one.*

Because in the end, the doctor the world needs is not the one who knows everything. But the one who *remains steady, clear, and responsible—in a world that is constantly changing.*

Epilogue

The Patient Returns

Somewhere along the journey, the patient disappeared.

Not physically. But conceptually.

They were replaced by reports, parameters, and protocols. By case sheets, scan images, and diagnostic labels. The conversation shifted from *"What is happening to this person?"* to *"What is this condition?"*

The system became efficient. But something essential was lost.

The person behind the disease.

And yet, the patient never truly left.

They were always present—in the hesitation before a diagnosis is spoken, in the silence after a difficult explanation, in the questions that are not asked but deeply felt.

They were present in the family waiting outside, in the financial worries quietly carried, in the fear of uncertainty that no report can capture.

The patient was always there. They were simply not fully seen.

This book began with a disturbance.

A recognition that medicine, while advancing in knowledge, was gradually narrowing in perception. That doctors, shaped by intense training and demanding systems, were becoming efficient processors of illness—but sometimes at the cost of human connection.

Not by intention. But by adaptation.

And now, it returns to a simple realization:

The patient must return to the center of medicine.

Not as an idea. But as a presence.

A presence that reminds the doctor that every condition exists within a life. That every decision affects more than the body. That every interaction carries weight beyond the clinical outcome.

When the patient returns, medicine expands again.

Science continues to guide decisions—but awareness shapes how those decisions are applied.

The disease is treated with precision. The person is engaged with understanding.

This is not a rejection of modern medicine.

It is its completion.

Technology, systems, and protocols are essential. They provide structure, scalability, and accuracy. But they must operate within a broader awareness—one that keeps the human dimension visible.

Otherwise, efficiency becomes isolation.

For the doctor, this return is not about doing more.

It is about seeing more.

Seeing the patient not only as a case, but as a participant. Not only as a receiver of treatment, but as a human navigating uncertainty.

This shift does not require additional time—it requires attention.

And attention changes everything.

For society, this return also brings responsibility.

To understand that doctors operate within constraints. That not every outcome can be controlled. That medicine is not a guarantee—it is a guided process.

Trust must be mutual. Understanding must be shared.

When both sides move toward awareness, something changes.

The consultation becomes a dialogue. The decision becomes a shared path. The outcome, whatever it may be, becomes easier to carry.

Because it is understood.

In the end, medicine does not regain its meaning through complexity.

It regains it through clarity.

Through the ability to treat disease with science—accurately, rigorously, and responsibly.

And to treat humans with awareness—respectfully, attentively, and honestly.

Because the future of medicine will not be defined only by how advanced it becomes.

But by whether, in that advancement, it remembers the simplest truth:

The patient was never just a case. And the doctor was never just a role.

When both are seen clearly, medicine finds its meaning again.

Closing Note

I did not write this book to conclude anything.

If anything, it has only made one thing clearer to me—that medicine, like every other serious human endeavor, is not a finished system. It is a living process, constantly shaped by people, pressure, progress, and perception.

And in that process, something essential is always at risk of being overlooked.

While writing this, I was not thinking as a doctor.

I was thinking as someone who observes systems.

How they evolve. How they stabilize. How they distort over time—not by intention, but by adaptation.

Medicine is no different.

It has not lost its meaning suddenly. It has been adjusting—quietly, continuously—to the demands placed on it.

And in that adjustment, the balance has shifted.

I have great respect for those who practice this profession.

Not in a symbolic or exaggerated way, but in a practical sense.

To work daily with uncertainty, to make decisions that carry weight, to function under pressure that does not pause—that requires a level of discipline and endurance that few professions demand.

At the same time, respect cannot prevent reflection.

In fact, it demands it.

This book does not attempt to correct medicine.

That would be unrealistic.

It does not attempt to define what a doctor should be.

That would be limiting.

It only attempts to bring attention to what is already happening.

To make visible the patterns that have become normal.

To create a moment of pause within a fast-moving system.

If you are a doctor, you already know more than this book can tell you.

What you may not always get is the space to observe how you are practicing.

That is what this book tries to offer.

Not answers.

But awareness.

If you are a patient, you may find parts of this book validating, and parts of it challenging.

That is intentional.

Because this system does not function through one side alone.

It is an interaction.

And interaction always carries shared responsibility.

I do not expect agreement.

I do not expect change.

But I do believe in observation.

Because once something is seen clearly, it cannot be unseen.

And that is where change—if it happens—begins.

Medicine will continue to evolve.

Systems will become more advanced. Technology will become more integrated. Processes will become more efficient.

That is inevitable.

What is not guaranteed is whether awareness will grow at the same pace.

And that is where the individual matters.

In the end, this book is not about medicine alone.

It is about how any profession—no matter how noble, complex, or advanced—can slowly drift away from its core if awareness is not maintained.

And how it can return—not through revolution, but through small, conscious alignment.

If this book has made you pause—even briefly—

then it has done enough.

— Sandeep

A doctor is not just a role within a system, but a human being functioning inside it.

A Note to Doctors

This book was written with you in mind.

Not as an outsider looking in, but as an observer trying to understand what your profession has become—and what it is becoming.

There is no denial of what it takes to become a doctor.

Years of discipline. Relentless competition. Exposure to suffering at an age when most are still understanding life itself.

By the time you enter practice, you are not just trained—you are shaped.

Your thinking is sharper. Your responses are faster. Your emotional engagement is measured.

This is not a flaw. It is a necessary adaptation.

But adaptation has a quiet side effect.

What begins as a way to survive the profession can slowly become the way you live within it.

Detachment becomes habit. Efficiency becomes default. Interaction becomes structured.

And without realizing it, the space between doctor and patient widens.

Not intentionally. But gradually.

This book does not question your knowledge.

It does not undermine your effort.

And it certainly does not ignore the constraints under which you work—time pressure, system demands, legal risks, administrative load.

These are real.

And they shape your decisions every day.

At the same time, there is another reality.

Patients still arrive with expectations that go beyond treatment. They look for clarity, reassurance, and trust.

When that expectation is not met, frustration grows. When frustration grows, trust weakens. And when trust weakens, the entire system becomes unstable.

You stand at the center of this tension.

Between system and patient. Between efficiency and engagement. Between knowledge and perception.

This position is not easy.

But it is significant.

The intention of this book is not to add pressure.

It is to bring awareness.

To highlight the small shifts that occur over time. To make visible what often goes unnoticed.

Not so that you change everything. But so that you see clearly.

Because clarity changes practice.

A small adjustment in how you listen, how you explain, how you respond under pressure—

can alter the entire experience for the patient.

And for you.

This is not about returning to an idealized version of medicine.

It is about practicing consciously within the reality you are already in.

Using systems—but not becoming them. Maintaining detachment—but not losing connection. Working efficiently—but not reducing interaction to a transaction.

You do not need to become a different doctor.

You need to become a more aware one.

If at any point while reading this book you felt challenged, uncomfortable, or even disagreed—that is not a problem.

That is engagement.

And engagement is where reflection begins.

There is no expectation that you will agree with everything written here.

But if you pause—once in a while—to observe your own practice a little more closely,

then this book has served its purpose.

Because medicine does not change through policy alone.

It changes through the way it is practiced—one interaction at a time.

And that remains in your control.

This book does not define what a doctor should be.

It simply asks you to define it—consciously.

Within your reality.

Within your system.

Within your practice.

And in doing so, perhaps restore something that was never lost—only overlooked.

The presence of the patient. And the awareness of the doctor.

A Note to Patients

This book has spoken extensively to doctors.

It is only fair that it speaks to you as well.

In moments of illness, vulnerability increases.

Uncertainty creates anxiety. Pain demands immediate attention. And in that state, the doctor becomes the center of expectation.

You expect clarity. You expect care. You expect certainty.

These expectations are natural.

But they are not always aligned with reality.

A doctor is not a machine that produces guaranteed outcomes.

Medicine is not an exact science in the way it often appears from the outside. It is a structured attempt to understand, manage, and influence complex biological processes—many of which remain uncertain.

Even with the best knowledge and intent, outcomes can vary.

This is not negligence. This is the nature of medicine.

Doctors operate within constraints that are often invisible.

Limited time per patient. Administrative and legal pressures. Resource limitations in many settings. Continuous exposure to illness, urgency, and responsibility.

These factors influence how they communicate, how they prioritize, and how they function.

At times, what appears as indifference may be fatigue. What feels like distance may be a protective response.

This does not justify poor behavior.

But it explains the environment in which behavior occurs.

At the same time, trust cannot be one-sided.

A healthy medical interaction requires participation.

Ask questions. Seek clarity. Share complete information. Express concerns—but with understanding.

The doctor is responsible for guiding. But you are responsible for engaging.

There is also a growing tendency to evaluate doctors only through outcomes.

If the result is favorable, trust increases. If not, doubt emerges.

This is a fragile way to judge a profession.

Because outcomes are influenced by multiple factors—timing, condition severity, biological variability, and response to treatment.

The process matters as much as the result.

Respect must also be mutual.

Doctors must respect patients as individuals—not just as cases.

But patients must also respect doctors as professionals—not as service providers who can be pressured, negotiated, or blamed beyond reason.

A system built on mistrust weakens both sides.

It is important to recognize that medicine is not a transaction.

It is an interaction.

One where knowledge meets vulnerability. One where decisions carry weight beyond the moment. One where communication can influence not just treatment—but experience.

This does not mean you should accept everything without question.

But questioning must be constructive—not confrontational.

Understanding must accompany expectation.

There will be doctors who meet your expectations.

There will be those who do not.

Just as in any profession.

But generalizing the entire system based on individual experiences only deepens the gap.

And that gap harms everyone.

If this book asks doctors to be more aware,

it also asks you to be more informed.

To see the doctor not only as an authority figure, but as a human being operating within a demanding system.

When both sides recognize this,

something changes.

Communication improves. Trust strengthens. Decisions become clearer.

Even difficult outcomes become easier to accept—because they are understood.

The goal is not perfection.

It is alignment.

Because the future of healthcare does not depend only on better technology or better systems.

It depends on better interactions.

Between doctor and patient.

Between expectation and reality.

Between science and understanding.

And that begins not with demands,

but with awareness.

A Note to Youngsters

Doctors and Medical Students

You are entering one of the most demanding professions in the world.

Not just academically. But psychologically.

Not just intellectually. But emotionally.

At this stage, your focus is clear.

Exams.

Concepts.

Clinical exposure.

Performance.

You are learning to recognize patterns, interpret data, and respond quickly. You are trained to think in structured ways, to prioritize efficiency, and to handle pressure.

All of this is necessary.

But there is something equally important that is rarely taught.

How to remain a doctor without losing yourself in becoming one.

The system will shape you.

Long hours will test your patience. Hierarchy will influence your confidence. Repetition will affect your sensitivity. Exposure to suffering will challenge your emotional balance.

Over time, you will adapt.

That adaptation will make you stronger.

But it can also make you rigid.

In the beginning, you will feel everything.

Every patient will seem important. Every case will feel intense. Every interaction will stay with you.

Gradually, that intensity will reduce.

This is natural.

You cannot carry every experience deeply and continue functioning.

So you will learn to detach.

Detachment is necessary.

But learn to control it.

Do not let it become your default state.

If you lose the ability to feel completely, you will protect yourself—but you will also distance yourself from the very purpose of your profession.

Balance matters.

You will also notice something else.

Speed will be rewarded.

You will be appreciated for handling more cases, making quicker decisions, and functioning efficiently within the system.

This is important.

But do not let speed replace understanding.

A fast doctor is useful. A clear doctor is effective.

There will be moments when you feel pressure to conform.

To follow what others are doing. To accept practices without questioning. To prioritize convenience over clarity.

Be careful in these moments.

Not everything that is common is correct.

At the same time, do not become idealistic in a way that ignores reality.

You will face constraints—time, infrastructure, patient load, administrative demands.

You cannot change everything.

But you can decide how you function within it.

Develop one habit early:
Pause before you conclude.
Even if it is for a few seconds.
That pause will allow you to:

- think clearly
- observe more
- avoid mechanical responses

Over time, this small habit will define your decision-making.

Communication is not a secondary skill.

It is part of treatment.

How you explain, how you listen, how you respond—these influence patient trust and cooperation as much as medication does.

Learn to communicate early.

Not perfectly. But consciously.

You will also make mistakes.

Every doctor does.

What matters is not the mistake—but how you respond to it.

Do you reflect? Do you adjust? Do you learn?

Or do you ignore and move forward without awareness?

Your response will shape your growth.

Do not build your identity only around being a doctor.

Maintain space for yourself outside the profession.

Your thinking, your relationships, your perspective on life—these will influence how you practice more than you realize.

A doctor who remains grounded as a person makes better decisions as a professional.

There will be times when you question your choice.

When fatigue, frustration, or system pressures feel overwhelming.

In those moments, do not look for motivation.

Look for clarity.

Why are you here? What does your role mean to you?

That clarity will stabilize you more than any external encouragement.

You are entering a system that is complex and evolving.

You will not control it.

But you will contribute to it.

Every interaction you have will shape how medicine is experienced by others.

You do not need to become a perfect doctor.

You need to become an aware one.

If you can preserve that awareness—through training, through pressure, through time—

then you will not just survive this profession.

You will practice it with clarity.

And that will make all the difference.

Key Reflections

From the Book

A patient is not a case. A case is only a tool—useful, necessary, but incomplete without the person it represents.

Clinical thinking simplifies reality. It must. But reality is always larger than the clinical frame, and what is simplified should never be mistaken for what is complete.

Detachment protects the doctor. It allows clarity, speed, and survival in demanding conditions. But when it goes unobserved, it quietly becomes distance—from the patient, and sometimes from the purpose of the profession itself.

Efficiency strengthens systems. It allows medicine to function at scale. Yet without awareness, efficiency can reduce interaction to a transaction, where the process is completed but the experience remains unattended.

Medical training sharpens intelligence. It builds precision, discipline, and analytical strength. But in doing so, it can also narrow perception—focusing on what is measurable while overlooking what is experienced.

A diagnosis explains a condition. It brings structure to uncertainty. But it does not explain the person living through that condition—their fear, their context, their expectations.

Trust is not built through expertise alone. It is built through clarity, consistency, and conduct—through how knowledge is applied and communicated.

The system provides structure. It organizes practice, reduces variability, and enables scale. But within that structure, it is the doctor who provides judgment.

Protocols guide decisions. They offer direction and safety. But they do not replace thinking. They are tools, not substitutes for awareness.

A fast doctor is useful. In a high-pressure environment, speed matters. But a clear doctor is effective—because clarity ensures that speed does not come at the cost of understanding.

Communication is not an addition to treatment. It is part of treatment. What is explained, how it is explained, and when it is explained all influence the outcome of care.

Patients arrive with biology and experience. Treating one without the other creates incomplete care. Both must be acknowledged for medicine to remain meaningful.

Uncertainty is not a weakness of medicine. It is a fundamental condition of it. Recognizing this does not reduce confidence—it strengthens honesty.

Outcomes are influenced by many factors—timing, biology, response, and context. But the process remains within control. And it is within the process that responsibility lies.

A good decision, if poorly communicated, creates doubt. A difficult decision, when clearly explained, creates trust.

Burnout is not only about workload. It is about prolonged misalignment—between what one does and how one understands it.

Repetition creates efficiency. It builds familiarity and speed. But if left unobserved, it can also create indifference.

Respect in medicine cannot be one-sided. It must exist between doctor and patient, as a shared understanding of roles and responsibilities.

Medicine is not practiced in isolation. It operates within a dynamic system of people, pressures, expectations, and constraints.

A doctor is not just a role within a system. A doctor is a human being functioning inside that system—and that distinction matters.

The profession demands responsibility. But it does not justify the loss of awareness. Responsibility and awareness must coexist.

Small shifts in behavior, repeated over time, reshape the entire practice. Not suddenly, but gradually.

The quality of interaction often defines the quality of experience—regardless of outcome.

Authority in medicine is given. Society grants it. But responsibility must be chosen—consciously, repeatedly.

The doctor stands between knowledge and uncertainty, navigating both. And that navigation requires awareness, not just expertise.

Systems influence behavior. They shape how decisions are made. But awareness regulates that influence.

A patient does not remember only what was prescribed. They remember how they were treated—how they were spoken to, how they were understood.

Clarity reduces conflict. Assumption increases it.

Medicine becomes mechanical when thinking is replaced by routine. And routine, if left unexamined, becomes habit.

A stable doctor creates a stable interaction. A fragmented doctor creates confusion—even when knowledge is correct.

The role of a doctor is not only to treat disease. It is to guide experience—through uncertainty, decision, and outcome.

Awareness is not an added skill. It is the foundation that holds all skills together.

The profession evolves. Technology advances. Systems change. But the core responsibility does not.

Medicine does not lose its meaning suddenly. It fades gradually—through small, unnoticed compromises.

And it regains meaning in the same way—through conscious alignment.

Because in the end, the patient was never just a case. And the doctor was never just a role.

Reflection Prompts for Practice

These are not questions to be answered once. They are prompts to revisit—quietly, honestly, and without pressure. Not at the end of a day, but in the middle of practice. Not for evaluation, but for awareness.

1. **When did I last listen without interrupting?** Not waiting to respond. Not filtering information. Just listening.
2. **Am I treating the condition—or understanding the situation?** Is my focus limited to diagnosis, or does it include the patient's context?
3. **Did I explain—or did I instruct?** Was the patient part of the decision, or simply the receiver of it?
4. **What am I prioritizing right now—speed or clarity?** And is that priority appropriate for this moment?
5. **Am I responding to the disease—or to the anxiety around it?** Often, what the patient needs first is not treatment, but understanding.
6. **Where did I assume instead of asking?** Assumptions save time. Questions create accuracy.
7. **Am I following the protocol—or thinking through it?** Is my decision active or automatic?
8. **Did I notice the person—or only the presentation?** A symptom is visible. A person is present.
9. **How did I communicate uncertainty?** Did I avoid it, or did I handle it with clarity?
10. **Was my detachment controlled—or habitual?** Did it

serve the situation, or distance me unnecessarily?

11. **Did I carry frustration from one interaction into another?** Or did I reset consciously?
12. **Where did I feel rushed—and why?** Was it system pressure, or internal urgency?
13. **Did I make space for questions—or close the interaction early?** Sometimes clarity is left unspoken because time feels limited.
14. **Am I practicing medicine—or managing workflow?** The difference is subtle, but significant.
15. **What did this interaction teach me?** Not academically, but practically.
16. **Did I act according to my standard—or adjust to convenience?** And if I adjusted, was it justified?
17. **How would I experience this interaction if I were the patient?** A simple shift in perspective can reveal a lot.
18. **What am I carrying from this day—and do I need to?** Not everything needs to be held beyond the moment.
19. **Am I becoming more clear—or more mechanical over time?** Repetition can build mastery—or reduce awareness.
20. **If I continue practicing this way, what kind of doctor will I become?** Not tomorrow, but over years.

These prompts are not meant to slow you down. They are meant to keep you aligned while moving fast.

Because in modern medicine, speed is inevitable. But awareness is a choice.

Acknowledgements

This book did not begin as a plan.

It began as a conversation.

An honest, slightly uncomfortable discussion with an old friend—shaped by his experiences, his frustrations, and his expectations from the medical profession. That conversation did not end that day. It stayed, evolved, and eventually found its way into these pages.

For that, I am grateful.

To the doctors—

Not just for what you do, but for what you endure.

This book questions certain patterns within the profession, but it does not ignore the effort behind it. The years of study, the long hours, the constant responsibility, and the pressure to make decisions that carry real consequences—these are not small things.

If this book challenges you, it is because your role matters.

To the patients—

Most of whom will never read this book, yet remain central to it.

Every interaction, every expectation, every moment of uncertainty you bring into the system is what gives medicine its meaning. You are not passive recipients of care—you are the reason care exists.

Your presence shaped the thinking behind this work.

To my students—

Who ask questions without hesitation.

Who challenge explanations. Who observe beyond what is taught.

Teaching has always been more than delivering concepts. It has been a continuous process of understanding how people think, react, and engage.

Many of the reflections in this book come from those interactions.

To the system—

With all its complexity, strengths, and limitations.

This book does not stand outside it. It observes from within its influence. The pressures, structures, and constraints that define modern medicine are not ignored—they are part of the reality this book addresses.

And finally, to the reader—

Whether you agreed, disagreed, or paused at certain points.

Engagement matters more than agreement.

If at any moment this book made you stop and observe your own perspective—on medicine, on doctors, on patients, or on systems—then it has fulfilled its purpose.

This book is not a conclusion.

It is part of an ongoing conversation.

One that continues beyond these pages—in practice, in interaction, and in the choices made every day within the field of medicine.

About the Author

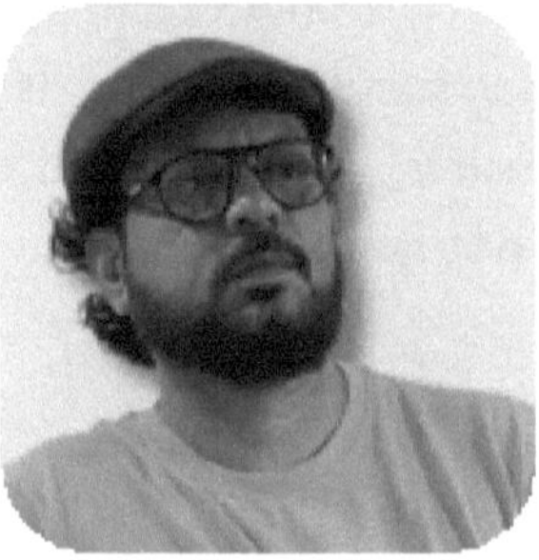

Sandeep J. Chavan is an engineer turned physics educator, independent researcher, and prolific author whose work spans science, human behavior, systems thinking, and philosophy.

With a background rooted in physics and years of experience teaching students at a fundamental level, he has developed a distinct approach that connects observation, interaction, and consequence across disciplines. His work often challenges conventional frameworks while offering simpler, more integrated ways of understanding complex realities.

He is the creator of the Universal Energy Dynamics (UED) framework, an attempt to unify concepts of energy, intelligence, human behavior, and system interactions under a single perspective. Through this lens, he explores not only physical phenomena, but also social systems, decision-making, and professional roles.

Over the years, he has authored numerous books across diverse domains—including physics, psychology, geopolitics, and reflective non-fiction—building what he refers to as the *Chavanian Ecosystem*, a connected body of work designed to make knowledge accessible, practical, and thought-provoking.

In this book, he brings the same lens to medicine—not as a clinician, but as an observer of systems and human behavior—offering a structured reflection on how doctors, patients, and healthcare systems interact in the modern world.

His writing is known for its clarity, directness, and ability to provoke thought without relying on complexity.

He continues to teach, write, and develop ideas that aim to bridge the gap between knowledge and awareness.

Further Reading

From the Chavanian Ecosystem

The ideas explored in this book do not exist in isolation.

They are part of a broader body of work that examines human behavior, systems, intelligence, and the deeper dynamics that shape how we think, decide, and interact.

The following books extend this discussion beyond medicine—into the mind, behavior, and systems that influence how medicine is practiced and experienced.

The 7 Psychological Wastes, A structured exploration of mental overload, decision fatigue, and hidden patterns that reduce clarity and efficiency—highly relevant in high-pressure professions like medicine.

The Active Mind, An in-depth look at how the mind reacts, processes, and adapts under pressure, offering insight into both patient behavior and clinical decision-making.

Soul Reframed: Energy, Mind, and the Architecture of Life, A structured perspective on consciousness, identity, and the internal experience of being human—useful for understanding suffering beyond biology.

Subconsciousness: The Chosen Disconnection, Explores how individuals disconnect from reality under stress, denial, or fear—directly applicable to patient responses and behavioral patterns.

Death: The Disconnection, A reflection on death as more than a biological event, addressing the experiential and psychological dimensions doctors encounter in practice.

Compare to Accept, Examines how comparison shapes perception, expectation, and dissatisfaction—useful for understanding both patient expectations and professional stress.

Universal Skill, Focuses on the ability to choose the right response in dynamic situations, a critical capability for effective decision-making in medicine.

The Untold Story of Intelligence and Mind, A foundational work on intelligence, awareness, and perception, expanding understanding beyond conventional clinical frameworks.

Chavanism: From Self to Civilization, A broader perspective on how individuals and systems evolve, stabilize, and distort—offering insight into the larger healthcare ecosystem.

The Mind That Won't Stop, A practical exploration of anxiety, overthinking, and internal noise—common experiences in both patients and medical professionals.

These works are part of the **Chavanian Ecosystem**—an interconnected body of ideas designed to move from isolated knowledge toward integrated understanding.

Because clarity in one domain often begins with awareness in another.

Disclaimer

This book is a work of reflective non-fiction intended to explore the dynamics of medical practice, doctor–patient interaction, and the broader healthcare system.

It is not a medical textbook, clinical manual, or professional guideline.

The content presented here does not provide medical advice, diagnosis, or treatment recommendations. It is not intended to replace formal medical education, clinical training, or professional judgment.

Doctors and medical professionals are advised to rely on established clinical guidelines, institutional protocols, and their own expertise while making medical decisions.

The perspectives in this book are observational and analytical in nature. They are based on the author's understanding of human behavior, systems, and professional environments, and are intended to encourage reflection—not to prescribe specific actions.

While every effort has been made to present ideas responsibly, the author does not assume responsibility for any decisions, actions, or outcomes arising from the interpretation or application of the content in this book.

This book does not intend to generalize, criticize, or misrepresent any individual, institution, or group within the medical profession. Any resemblance to specific individuals or situations is unintentional and coincidental.

Healthcare is a complex, evolving system influenced by multiple factors, including infrastructure, policy, resource availability, and individual circumstances. The discussions in this book acknowledge this complexity and are not intended to oversimplify or reduce it.

Readers are encouraged to engage with the material thoughtfully and interpret it within their own professional, personal, and situational context.

The purpose of this book is reflection.

Any insight or change that arises from it is the responsibility of the reader's own awareness and judgment.

Don't miss out!

Visit the website below and you can sign up to receive emails whenever Sandeep Chavan publishes a new book. There's no charge and no obligation.

https://books2read.com/r/B-A-EPGPC-IQIDJ

BOOKS 2 READ

Connecting independent readers to independent writers.

Did you love *When the Patient Became a Case*? Then you should read *What Collapses Your Reputation*[1] by Sandeep Chavan!

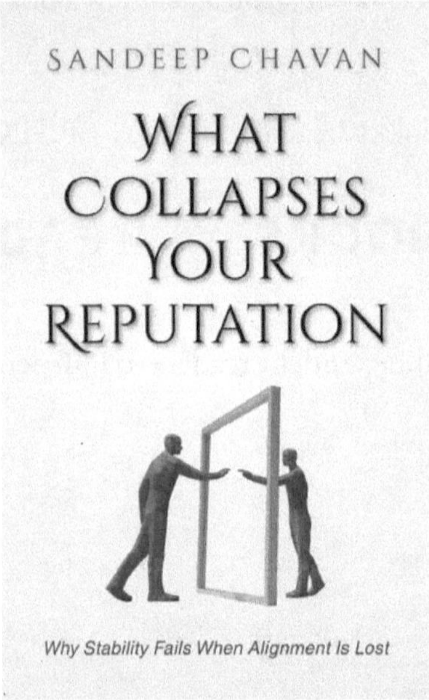

[2]

Reputation is rarely lost the way people imagine.

It does not collapse through scandal, public failure, or obvious mistakes. More often, it collapses quietly—while everything still appears intact.

In *What Collapses Your Reputation*, Sandeep Chavan explores reputation not as an achievement to be protected, but as a social consequence that behaves predictably when alignment is present—and fails silently when it is asked to do too much.

Through a series of narrative-driven case studies—a reputed doctor on a long train journey, a former MLA navigating life after electoral loss, and a respected corporate manager unraveling over

1. https://books2read.com/u/mZy8JR

2. https://books2read.com/u/mZy8JR

tea—the book traces a common but rarely named pattern. Across professions, power levels, and social settings, reputation remains visible while ease disappears. Respect persists, yet something essential tightens.

This is not a self-help book. It offers no advice, techniques, or motivational prescriptions. Instead, it observes how modern life quietly shifts from living to managing, from responding to defending, and from being to maintaining.

The book reveals how reputation collapses not when it is attacked from the outside, but when it is overloaded from within—when it moves from being an effect of alignment to a substitute for it. As reputation becomes central, movement narrows. Control replaces trust. Stability hardens into rigidity.

Written in a calm, literary, and accessible style, *What Collapses Your Reputation* avoids the vocabulary of conventional psychology and self-improvement. It speaks to professionals, leaders, thinkers, and readers who sense that life has become heavier despite everything "working."

This book does not tell you what to change.It shows you what is already happening.

For anyone who has felt the quiet pressure of holding things together, this book offers clarity—not correction.

Read more at https://www.sandeepjchavan.com/.

www.ingramcontent.com/pod-product-compliance
Lightning Source LLC
LaVergne TN
LVHW100250210926
848480LV00003B/887